AROMATHERAPY and ESSENTIAL OILS for HEALING

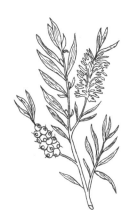

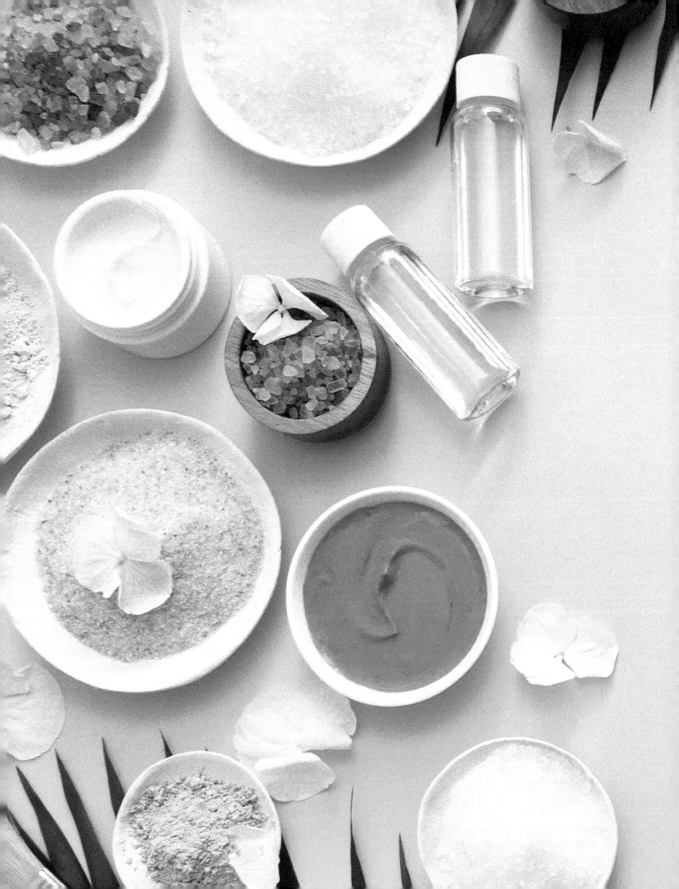

AROMATHERAPY and ESSENTIAL OILS for HEALING

120 Remedies to Restore Mind, Body, and Spirit

AMBER ROBINSON

ROCKRIDGE
PRESS

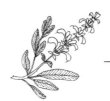

To my husband and sons, who have supported me
on my journey every step of the way.

CONTENTS

Part Two: Remedies for Healing and Prevention

Introduction

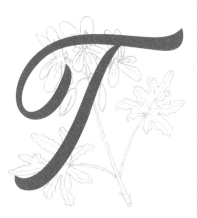

The first time I realized the full healing potential of essential oils was when I came down with a nasty cold. I was experiencing a lot of congestion that resulted in painful sinus headaches. At the time, I wasn't as knowledgeable about essential oils, but I found them intriguing and had purchased several from a company a friend recommended. I diffused a combination of clove, cinnamon, and rosemary essential oils and was surprised when I felt remarkably better within a day. My congestion broke up and I could breathe again. My headaches subsided, and the pressure that caused them was gone. It was then I knew I was on to something.

My interest in essential oils grew from there, and I realized what little I knew about essential oils was not enough. I had to find out more. Everything I had learned came from a friend who sold essential oils. After taking steps to become formally educated in aromatherapy, I began to learn that what I thought I knew was not entirely accurate. I had been applying essential oils incorrectly and using the wrong (and potentially unsafe) essential oils around my children. This is one reason I am passionate about educating others on proper essential oil usage. Many of the tips and tricks people are given are not only ineffective but can also be downright dangerous. It is my aim to help others feel empowered to use essential oils in a way that is not just safe but also increases the effectiveness of the oils being used.

My love of essential oils blossomed to the point that I decided to create my own, using steam distillation. I began growing plants on my farm and creating unusual and rare essential oils. Intimately learning what goes into creating essential oils has shown me that these oils are more precious than most people realize. When I learned how essential oils are made, it didn't take long to realize that they are a kind of treasure. Every drop is hard-earned. One dram of essential oil is the result of hours of toil: early-morning walks around the farm to collect huge baskets of dew-covered flowers, the tedious filling of the still, the hours-long process of letting the water boil at just the right temperature to extract the oils, the careful separation of the essential oils from the hydrosol to make sure I get each drop. All this effort goes into making one small bottle of essential oil, and most people take it for granted. When you realize the value of each drop, you will also be able to grasp just how effective these concentrated and powerful oils can be when used properly.

Today, I use essential oils in many ways. I have perfected recipes through the years and have experienced their effectiveness firsthand. I am very proud to be able to share these recipes with you. This book covers what you need to know about essential oils to get started and provides helpful remedies that work. Soak up the valuable information and enjoy the remedies!

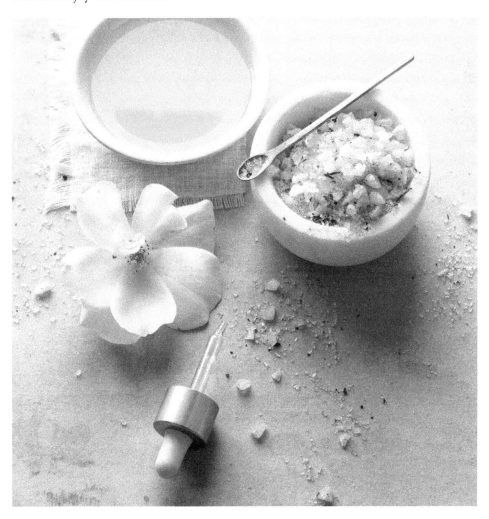

Part One

The Healing Power of Aromatherapy

In the first part of this book, you will learn about the healing powers of essential oils in more depth. This section empowers you with an understanding of the history of aromatherapy, how essential oils are made, how they work in the body, how to choose oils wisely, how to use oils properly, and how to practice aromatherapy using a safe and mindful approach. You will learn everything you need to get the most out of each essential oil you work with and become more confident when working with oils.

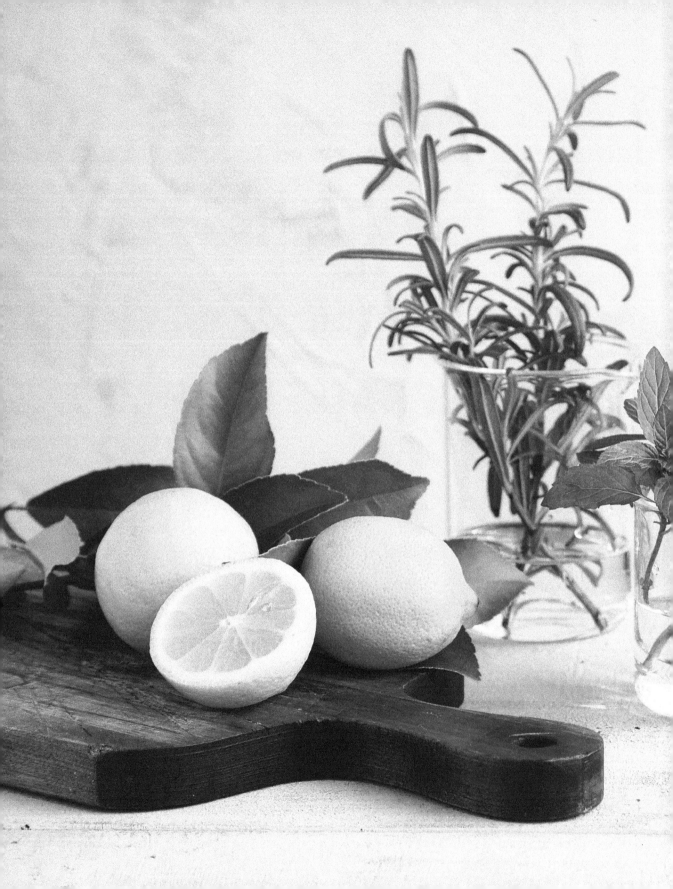

1

WHAT IS AROMATHERAPY?

Welcome to the world of healing with aromatherapy and essential oils! In this chapter, I will explain the basics of essential oils and aromatherapy. Whether you are new to essential oils or have been using them for some time, it is helpful to understand the history of aromatherapy, the science behind this ancient practice, and the evolution of essential oils as they are known today.

History

Essential oils have been used since ancient times to help heal the body and mind. The ancient Egyptians are often credited with being the first to use essential oils. They prized essential oils for more than just their wonderful aromas: The fragrant oils were an integral part of the embalming process, and also used in spiritual and relaxation practices and for cosmetic purposes.

Eventually, the ancient Greeks began experimenting with essential oils, using them in a similar manner to the Egyptians for healing and relaxation. The Greeks also heavily incorporated essential oils and herbs into their medicinal practices. The Greek physician Hippocrates was the first known physician to discuss the use of plant-based medicines in his practices.

The ancient Romans, in turn, adopted many of the healing techniques used by the Greeks and Egyptians. From there, the Persians are credited with advancing the technology used in distilling essential oils. A famous Persian physician, Avicenna, developed a special pipe for distillation. Before this, most aromatic substances were closer to floral water than oil. Later on, the Crusades led to the spread of aromatherapy throughout Europe.

The Uses of Aromatherapy

The art of aromatherapy has evolved over time. Discoveries and advancements in the scientific study of essential oils have revealed how they can help with myriad issues. Aromatherapy has a wide range of applications, including beauty, skin care, health, and even household uses such as cleaning and killing bacteria on surfaces. Some essential oils contain anti-aging properties, making them ideal for use in serums for aging skin. Others can kill germs and bacteria and are helpful in preventing the spread of pathogens that could cause illness. It is an exciting time to get into aromatherapy, as more and more studies are proving the therapeutic and practical uses of essential oils.

Aromatherapy for Healing

Aromatherapy is the combination of the ancient Greek words *arōma*, meaning "spice or sweet herb," and *therapeía*, meaning "healing." Of all the uses for essential oils, healing is the most prominent. From emotional to physical healing, essential oils can provide relief and enhance overall wellness.

One of the first scientific discoveries pertaining to the healing properties of essential oils was when a French chemist named René Maurice Gattefossé accidentally discovered that lavender essential oil could soothe and heal burns in the 1920s. He burned himself while working in his laboratory and decided to thrust his wounded hand into the nearest cold liquid he could find, which happened to be lavender oil. The pain and irritation from the burn subsided, and his hand healed remarkably well.

Over the years, studies have not only shown that lavender and other essential oils can be helpful for various physical ailments, but also demonstrated that essential oils can help with emotional issues. For example, bergamot essential oil can be great for oily and acne-prone skin but can also treat anxiety and depression. Lemon essential oil can help brighten the complexion and energize and uplift a tired mind.

What Are Essential Oils?

Essential oils are concentrated plant isolates created through various extraction methods that separate the oils from the rest of the plant material. The result of the distillation process is a highly aromatic and potent essential oil, or the "essence" of the plant itself. It usually takes a large amount of plant material to create a small amount of essential oil. For example, 22 pounds of rose petals yield just 5 milliliters of rose essential oil. (Rose petals are very light, so this is a lot of petals!) The plant material is exposed to steam or carbon dioxide (CO_2), depending on the extraction method. This helps release the oils from the plant. When the process is complete, hydrosol (plant-infused water) is usually left behind, with essential oils floating on top to be collected. Some of the most popular and common essential oils include clary sage, clove, eucalyptus, frankincense, geranium, grapefruit, lavender, lemon, lemongrass, patchouli, peppermint, Roman chamomile, rosemary, tea tree, and thyme. These oils, and others, are highlighted in essential oil profiles and recipes later in this book to help you gain a deeper knowledge of how to use them and the benefits they provide.

Extraction Methods

Three major extraction methods are used to collect essential oils. The first, oldest, and arguably most popular is steam distillation. This involves placing plant material in a flask above boiling water. As the steam travels through the plant material, it collects the essential oils. The steam then re-condenses into liquid as it travels through a condenser coil. It emerges from the still as hydrosol, or plant water. As this hydrosol collects in a container, essential oils begin to float on top. At the end of the steam distillation process, the essential oils are separated from the hydrosol. A variation is hydro distillation, which involves putting the plant material in the water instead of above it. The steam distillation process is fun to watch and has been around for a long time. However, it is not the most efficient method for collecting all of the potential oils.

Another method for extracting essential oils is called cold pressing. Cold pressing is mostly used for extracting citrus essential oils, which come from citrus peels. The peels are placed in a device that punctures them to release the oils. The device uses a centrifuge to separate the oils from the pulp and other liquid. This process is effective because it doesn't damage the plant material with heat like other extraction methods. The drawback to this process is that not all oils can be made this way: Only plants with peels can be used.

The final and most modern extraction method is CO_2 extraction. This method involves controlling the temperature and pressure in a chamber with plant material. The application of CO_2 acts as a solvent to help release the oils from the plants. This process is great for getting the most oils from a plant, resulting in much less waste than other extraction methods. However, it involves expensive machinery, and some argue that the use of this solvent can affect the quality of the yield.

The Science Behind It All

Essential oils have been found to be effective because they contain therapeutic constituents like terpenes, aldehydes, esters, and phenols that target specific issues. Because of advancements in technology (specifically, a device called a chromatograph), researchers have been able to break down essential oils to their individual constituents to determine exactly how and why they work to heal the body and mind.

One of these researchers, Otto Wallach, won the Nobel Prize in chemistry in 1910 for isolating aromatic organic compounds that he called terpenes. Sesquiterpenes, a kind of terpene found in chamomile and rose, have anti-inflammatory properties. Monoterpenes are found in differing amounts in almost every essential oil. Some essential oils high in monoterpenes include lavender, clary sage, and basil. These beneficial compounds have strong antimicrobial properties and help enhance mood.

Aldehydes, including citrusy oils like Melissa (lemon balm) and lemongrass, possess antifungal and disinfectant properties. Esters are another therapeutic constituent that can be antispasmodic and sedative. Lavender essential oil contains a type of ester called linalyl acetate. Other constituents, like phenols, have been shown to be antiseptic and antibacterial. Oils like cinnamon and clove contain phenols. Inhaling essential oils or using them topically allows these constituents to enter the body and promote healing.

What Can Essential Oils Do?

Because essential oils are the concentrated result of a large amount of plant material, they are highly potent and powerful when it comes to healing. This means that essential oils do not have to be used in large amounts to be effective. A little truly goes a long way. In many cases, simple inhalation can be effective for issues ranging from anxiety to respiratory issues. For example, inhaling eucalyptus essential oil can relieve congestion and sinus pressure. For anxiety, inhalation of lavender has been shown to reduce stress and promote relaxation.

There are times when a drop or two of certain essential oils works best topically. For example, a small amount of frankincense essential oil diluted in a carrier oil and applied to aging skin can help prevent wrinkles and promote skin elasticity and health. The potency of essential oils makes them perfect remedies for these conditions and others—and one bottle can last for years!

How to Use Essential Oils

There are several ways to use essential oils. The most popular method is direct inhalation. This is the way they were originally administered, hence the name "aroma" therapy. Our olfactory system works by identifying scent molecules, spurring the brain to react. Scent is strongly tied to memory and emotion, and certain aromas can evoke positive and negative emotions. When therapeutic constituents in essential oils interact with our olfactory nerves and brain, amazing things can happen, from memory enhancement to stress reduction. For example, an effective way to treat stress and anxiety is to place a few drops of lavender essential oil in a personal inhaler and inhale deeply.

Topical application is another popular method. When an essential oil is properly diluted and applied to an affected area, it can help bring relief and healing for issues ranging from skin rashes to scarring. Essential oils like frankincense oil have specific healing capabilities when applied topically. Frankincense has been shown in studies to possess antioxidant activity, thus promoting skin healing and clarity.

Essential oils can also be used via diffusion. With diffusion, essential oils are placed in an ultrasonic diffuser to be distributed throughout the atmosphere in a specific area. Ultrasonic diffusion allows the therapeutic constituents to mingle with water in the atmosphere. This allows for inhalation as well as air purification. Essential oils like clove oil contain antiviral constituents that have been shown to combat viruses when diffused in a small room.

NEBULIZING DIFFUSERS

Nebulizing diffusers are another type of essential oil diffuser. They work differently than ultrasonic diffusers because they do not require water. Nebulizing diffusers disperse essential oils directly into the atmosphere in the room. They tend to be more expensive than ultrasonic diffusers and use more oil. Use caution when running one of these diffusers around pets and children, as the oil concentration in the air will be much higher than if you were using an ultrasonic diffuser.

Essential Oils Today

Essential oils today are somewhat different than those used many years ago. This is largely because of advancements in extraction method technology. The oils available today are as potent and pure as ever.

It seems like essential oils are everywhere, so it's important to understand what separates good-quality essential oils from adulterated oils. An adulterated essential oil has been diluted with another substance, usually alcohol or another (much cheaper) oil. Be wary of purchasing essential oils at extremely cheap, discounted prices, as this is a sign they may be adulterated. In addition, avoid ordering oils online from large e-commerce stores because you never know what you will get or if it's a quality product. It's best to procure oils from trusted distributors or straight from the source, but by reading labels and purchasing from reputable local health stores with knowledgeable and trained staff, you'll be off to a great start.

READING THE LABEL

Most essential oils will have certain information on the bottle, such as the common name of the plant used, the Latin name of the plant used, the country of origin (where the plants came from), and which extraction method was used to obtain the oil. Knowing the common and Latin names of the plants is very important because this helps you distinguish between the species used to create the oil. Some species are more medicinal than others, and even if two plants are in the same family, they are likely not used for the same issues. For example, when purchasing cinnamon essential oil, you will have to look closely at the label to see whether the leaf or bark of the cinnamon tree is used. The leaf is much safer for young ones than the bark. Additionally, there are two popular types of cinnamon (Ceylon and Cassia), and Ceylon cinnamon is the most therapeutic. Knowing the differences is crucial from a practical perspective and for safety reasons. A good company will include the most thorough safety information possible on the label. For essential oil blends, look for the percentages of each oil used. Some companies omit this information, which can be dangerous when dealing with oils that are known to cause skin sensitization or irritation.

Grades and Purity

It won't take long when reading labels on essential oils to notice terms like "certified therapeutic grade" and "100 percent pure." Almost every essential oil on the market boasts these claims. However, the informed consumer must be aware that these terms do not mean much at all. In fact, there is no official third party that certifies an essential oil as "therapeutic grade" or "100 percent pure." The truth is that the company is certifying itself with these distinctions, so take this information with a grain of salt. One exception is any oil that is USDA-certified organic. These certifications come from the United States Department of Agriculture and require a company to go through many steps to obtain the certification.

Now that we've covered some of the basics of essential oils and aromatherapy, it is time to delve into the specifics of this practice. Chapter 2 goes into more detail about aromatherapy, as well as the healing properties and uses of different essential oils.

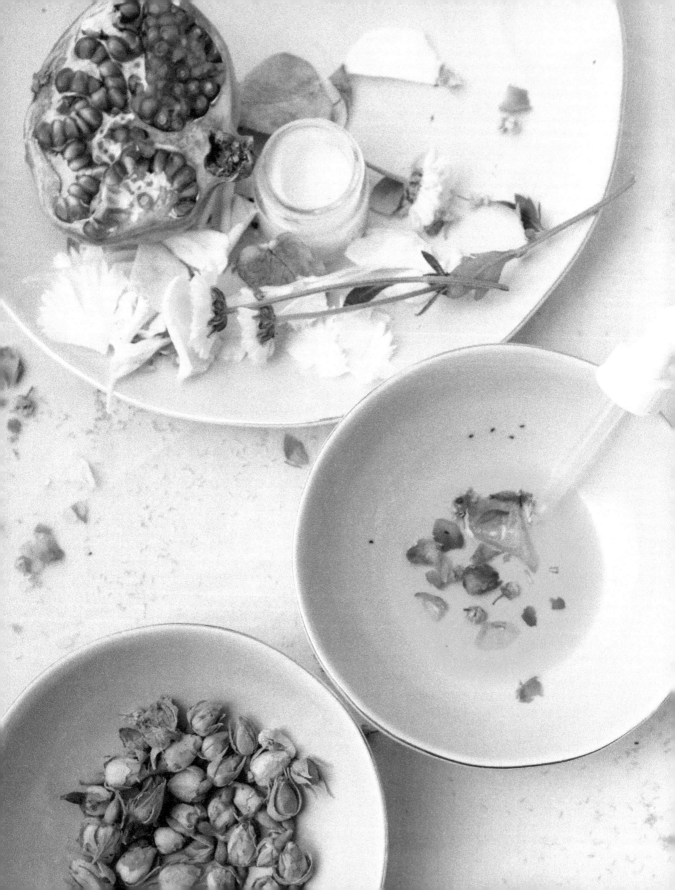

2

EMOTIONAL AND PHYSICAL HEALING

This chapter gets into the specifics of healing with aromatherapy. You'll learn how aromatherapy heals, what exactly it can heal, the basics of application, the importance of self-care, and some key terminology.

How Aromatherapy Heals

One of the most prominent ways aromatherapy can foster healing is by relieving stress and promoting relaxation. In our fast-paced, busy society, it seems as though everyone is operating at full capacity all the time. This constant state of activity and stimulation results in lots of stress and burnout.

Our adrenal glands, located on top of each kidney, are responsible for providing our bodies with the hormones necessary to help us deal with stress. Today, many people experience adrenal fatigue because of overstimulation and being constantly on the go. While it may be important to have an active lifestyle, the old adage "everything in moderation" is important to keep in mind. It can be hard for some people's adrenal glands to keep up with constant stress and activity. Adrenal fatigue can result in depression, dizziness, extreme fatigue, dark undereye circles, insomnia, joint pain, and a variety of other unwelcome symptoms.

This is where aromatherapy can really make a difference. A May 2019 study in *Neuroscience Letters* shows that lavender essential oil can reduce the effects of depression, especially when it's caused by adrenal hormone overproduction. This is great news for those looking for a tool to add to their self-care routine. The sedative and calming properties of essential oils like lavender interact with the olfactory system and the brain to help reduce stress. Reduced stress results in a healthier, happier person.

Stress doesn't just affect us mentally and emotionally; it can trigger physical problems like autoimmune disease flare-ups, weight gain, heart disease, and more. In addition to reducing stress via the olfactory system, aromatherapy heals when essential oils are applied topically by delivering compounds with antioxidant, anti-inflammatory, and antimicrobial effects that target issues ranging from burns to acne.

A Holistic Therapy

Aromatherapy makes a great addition to your holistic healing routine. The term *holistic* means looking at the body as a whole, rather than focusing on individual symptoms or parts. This concept is crucial when determining the approach to take to deal with various symptoms or issues. Mainstream health care often treats the symptoms of a larger issue, rather than trying to tackle the root of the problem. The holistic approach aims to treat the whole body, while attempting to find and treat the cause of the issue. This alternative healing approach can complement other types of healing, including Western medicine practices. Including aromatherapy in your a holistic healing approach gives you another tool for targeting your root problem.

Certifications and Professional Healing

A certification in aromatherapy is a great complement to professions such as massage therapy or social work. With the deeper knowledge of aromatherapy that comes with high-quality training, those who practice professionally can enhance their work, provide clients with top-notch care, and feel great knowing they are making a difference in the lives of the people they encounter each day.

In the United States, there aren't any degrees available in the field of aromatherapy, so anyone interested in becoming an aromatherapist must obtain a certification through a credible school or institution. These can be found by visiting the website of the National Association of Holistic Aromatherapy (NAHA). This association is a nonprofit institution "devoted to the holistic integration and education of aromatherapy into a wide range of complementary healthcare practices." It has the resources and information you need to get started, should you be interested in practicing aromatherapy at a professional level.

Aromatherapy and Acupuncture

Acupuncture is the practice of stimulating specific points on the body using very small needles. Some acupuncturists use aromatherapy in their practice by applying certain essential oils (instead of needles) to those points of the body in order to stimulate the area. Sometimes the oils are used in conjunction with the needles. A practitioner who combines aromatherapy with acupuncture should be a trained professional with a deep understanding of specific oil constituents, effects, and safety. When these techniques are used correctly, the experience can be especially healing.

Aromatherapy and Herbal Studies

Aromatherapy and herbal studies go hand in hand. Essential oils are the derivatives of plants, and herbalists are trained to understand the medicinal actions of plants and how to use them properly on a case-by-case basis. Most herbalists already have a very strong knowledge of the plants used to create oils and work with both essential oils and plants.

WHAT IF I WANT TO BECOME AN AROMATHERAPIST?

Becoming a certified aromatherapist begins with choosing a school that is right for you. Do you want to attend a brick-and-mortar school or an online school? The NAHA website has a list of NAHA-approved schools that prospective students can browse through (see Resources, page 193). There are many choices available. Ask the school questions like: Which levels of certification do you offer? Will instructors be readily available to answer any questions I may have?

According to NAHA, a level 1 certified aromatherapist has completed a minimum of 50 hours of training. This level of training is great for health professionals like nurses, herbalists, and massage therapists. In the 50 hours, a student must complete at least 20 essential oil profiles and five case studies, as well as learn about the history of aromatherapy, essential oil quality, methods of extraction, physiological effects of oils, how oils interact with the body physically and emotionally, basic oil chemistry, blend design, methods of application, safety, and legal issues concerning aromatherapy.

A NAHA level 2 aromatherapist must complete a minimum of 200 hours of curriculum, and a NAHA level 3 aromatherapist must complete a minimum of 300 hours of curriculum. More details on how to attain these distinctions through NAHA are available on the NAHA website, NAHA.org.

What Can Aromatherapy Help With?

From everyday skin care routines and stress reduction to providing relief from wasp stings and healing minor cuts and scrapes, essential oils come in handy for a wide range of home remedies. Aromatherapy can be employed for emotional healing from anxiety, nervousness, frustration, tension, and fear. It can also be used to aid in physical healing for pain, skin issues, gastrointestinal problems, and more. In addition, aromatherapy can be used as part of your beauty routine to promote clear skin and skin elasticity, and some essential oils even reduce the appearance of scars, dark circles, and stretch marks.

Physical Healing

When it comes to physical healing, essential oils can provide relief for a variety of physical ailments. Clary sage can help relieve menstrual cramps and provide PMS relief when applied externally to the lower abdomen. Chamomile essential oil has antispasmodic and pain-relieving properties that make it useful for the treatment of charley horses and body aches or muscle spasms. Patchouli essential oil is great for promoting the regeneration of skin cells, as well as healing dry, cracked skin. This is why it is part of skin care routines for aging and dry skin. There are so many benefits when it comes to what essential oils can do for physical healing.

Emotional Healing

In addition to healing physical ailments, aromatherapy can be also effective in treating issues like anxiety, depression, and insomnia. Lavender essential oil can reduce stress and symptoms of depression. Other essential oils like chamomile and orange can promote feelings of relaxation and calm while promoting feelings of positivity and optimism. Valerian root essential oil affects the central nervous system and helps the body fall asleep more efficiently. Essential oils can do amazing things to promote emotional health.

Healing Properties of Essential Oils

Essential oils can have many different healing properties. Some of the most common healing properties are antispasmodic (preventing bodily spasms), antibacterial (destroying bacteria), anti-inflammatory (preventing inflammation), antiviral (destroying viral pathogens), astringent (tightening tissues), carminative (helping with stomach issues), emollient (softening the skin), expectorant (helping the body get rid of excess mucus), sedative (calming), and uterine (healing to the uterus). You will find out more about these healing properties throughout this book.

Remedies

Using essential oils to create healing remedies is a central part of this book. A remedy is simply a formulation using one or more essential oils, as well as a carrier oil or other means of proper dilution, to create a targeted therapeutic treatment for a certain issue or ailment. The remedies in this book are cost-effective, using popular and common essential oils, and are great for beginners and experienced healers alike.

Application

Each remedy in this book specifies a method of application. Methods of application are important when trying to get the maximum benefits out of your precious essential oils. There are two application methods: topical application and inhalation.

Topical

Remedies that call for topical application will require proper dilution before they are applied. Depending on the remedy, it may require the diluted formulation to be applied topically to pulse points like the wrists, inner elbows, or neck. Some remedies will be more targeted in terms of topical application. For example, a remedy for gastrointestinal discomfort may require that you massage the blend into the abdomen in order to experience the best results. A remedy for menstrual cramping will usually require the blend to be massaged into the lower abdomen or uterine area.

Inhalation

Remedies that call for inhalation are often utilized via a personal inhaler. This method is simple: You drop the required amount of essential oils onto a wick or cotton ball and inhale for relief. Inhalation works best for emotional issues. It is also the preferred method if using aromatherapy around children or during pregnancy. Inhalation is a more cautious approach than topical application, given that the oils do not come into physical contact with the body.

Another type of inhalation is diffusion, when oils are added to an ultrasonic diffuser or similar device and distributed throughout the atmosphere. This type of inhalation is sometimes called atmospheric diffusion or atmospheric inhalation. Because this method affects everyone in the room where the diffusion is taking place, it's important to be respectful of others, especially children, as everyone reacts to oils differently.

Wellness Starts with Self-Care

According to the American Psychological Association, self-care is vitally important for our health and critical to prevent burnout, distress, and other emotional issues. Self-care can include setting aside time to relax or get more sleep, spend time with friends or family, or do something you enjoy. Centering yourself through these self-care practices is important to staying well physically, mentally, and emotionally.

Aromatherapy can enhance the benefits of your self-care practices. Whether it is scheduling a massage with a practitioner who works with essential oils or relaxing in a Healing Detox Bath Soak (page 117) to relax, incorporating aromatherapy in your self-care routine can help you heal from the negative effects of daily stress.

Beauty

Using essential oils for beauty and wellness can have a dramatic effect on both the outside and inside. The truth is that many commercial beauty products like deodorants, shampoos, lotions, creams, and soaps are filled with aluminum, parabens, synthetic fragrances, dyes, and sulfates that can affect our health in a serious way. Substituting these products with the natural remedies in this book means you can be confident you are not putting something unhealthy or harmful in or on your body. This is the very essence of self-care.

In addition, using aromatherapy in your beauty routine can help provide real healing, rather than simply masking an issue. Essential oils can be a great preventive treatment for all kinds of issues with the skin, hair, and nails.

Skin Care

Aromatherapy can heal, balance, and restore skin. Essential oils can treat acne, oily skin, dry skin, rashes, burns, cuts and scrapes, dark circles, stretch marks, and scarring; can treat and prevent wrinkles; and can improve skin tone and luster. Bergamot essential oil is a vibrant citrus essential oil perfect for controlling oily skin. Tea tree essential oil has been shown to help kill the bacteria responsible for creating acne and blackheads. Frankincense essential oil is a great choice for treating wrinkles, scarring, and aging skin because of its antioxidant activity. Other oils, such as lavender and chamomile, can help calm the skin and promote healthy skin tone.

Hair Care

As we age, our hair can become more prone to breakage and damage. This often escalates after childbirth, when hormones contribute to hair loss and brittleness. Some essential oils contain hair-strengthening properties and are great for nourishing and enriching hair follicles. Rosemary essential oil not only helps the hair shaft but can also improve circulation on the scalp, which can help encourage hair growth and health. Geranium essential oil can improve hair luster and health and is often used in commercial skin and hair products.

AROMATHERAPY LIKE A PRO

Want to talk about aromatherapy like an expert? Acquaint your-self with these terms to better understand various oils and their medicinal actions.

ABSOLUTE: an essential oil extracted by means of a chemical solvent

ANALGESIC: pain-relieving

ANTI-ALLERGENIC: relieves or reduces allergy symptoms

ANTIBACTERIAL: destroys the growth of bacteria

ANTIDEPRESSANT: helps relieve feelings of depression

ANTIFUNGAL: destroys the growth of fungi

ANTI-INFLAMMATORY: reduces inflammation

ANTIMICROBIAL: destroys the growth of microorganisms

ANTIOXIDANT: inhibits cellular oxidation

ANTISPASMODIC: prevents spasms or convulsions

ANTITUSSIVE: helps suppress coughs

ANTIVIRAL: destroys viruses

APHRODISIAC: sparks sexual desire

ASTRINGENT: tightens body tissues

BOTANICAL NAME: the Latin name given to a species of plant to distin-guish it from other plants that share the same common name

CARMINATIVE: relieves gas

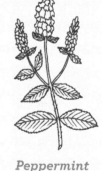

Peppermint

CARRIER OIL: a vegetable oil, derived from the fatty part of a plant, used to dilute an essential oil

CIRCULATORY: pertaining to the circulatory system or to circulation

COMMON NAME: the generic or conventional name given to a plant

DECONGESTANT: relieves congestion

DIGESTIVE: promotes digestion

DISINFECTANT: destroys bacteria that could cause infection

DIURETIC: promotes excretion of urine from the body

DRAM: a unit of measurement equaling ⅛ ounce

EMOLLIENT: softens or soothes the skin

EXPECTORANT: promotes expulsion of mucus and phlegm

FEBRIFUGE: helps reduce fever

HYDRATING: restores moisture

HYDROSOL: the plant-infused water byproduct of the essential oil distillation process

IMMUNOSTIMULANT: stimulates the immune system

NERVINE: helps calm the nerves

SEDATIVE: calming

UTERINE: relating to or affecting the uterus

Spa Treatments

One of the most enjoyable ways to use aromatherapy is for relaxation. Essential oils can be a great addition to your at-home spa treatments. Adding essential oils like lavender and clary sage to Epsom salts not only provides a lovely aroma but also enhances the therapeutic effects of a soothing bath. Add geranium or patchouli essential oil to bentonite clay to create a detoxifying and soothing clay mask that promotes glowing, healthy skin, or put a few drops in boiling water to create a nourishing facial steam treatment for pore cleansing and skin regeneration.

A HEALING SPACE

You don't need a ton of room to create your own healing station. Consider turning a corner of your house (the bathroom, your bedroom, or another private spot) into a place where you can retreat to relax. Add shelving to store your natural remedies for quick and easy access to your favorite treatments. A comfortable chair that allows you to elevate your feet can be great for unwinding at the end of a long day. Dim lighting, such as a Himalayan salt lamp, sets the perfect mood. (Make sure to keep the salt lamp away from pets, as they can be toxic to some animals.) An ultrasonic diffuser is another amazing accessory. Keep the decorations and clutter minimal, as this can trigger stress for many people. Imagine being able to come to your very own place, lit by the soft light of a therapeutic lamp, with the relaxing aromas of essential oils diffusing into the air around you, while you kick back in your chair enjoying your geranium clay mask. Close your eyes and take this quiet time to meditate on your favorite things. Even 20 minutes each day in a space like this can reduce stress and improve your mood.

Keep Yourself Well

Aromatherapy isn't just for treating specific problems, although it works great for many physical and emotional issues. It can also function as preventive medicine and part of your self-care routine. When you engage in self-care, you are actually contributing to your overall wellness by taking steps to reduce your stress levels. This is vital for maintaining your health on many levels.

Stay Balanced

Aromatherapy can help you feel balanced. Achieving balance can help you feel more optimistic about life, and help bring you into the moment. Staying balanced is pivotal. Imbalance, when left unchecked, can lead to difficulties with depression, anxiety, and poor health. Being grounded in everyday life means being in control of your emotions, as well as having the clarity to think and act as your best self.

Practice Self-Care

Creating self-care rituals can help prevent issues before they begin to manifest. Taking the time to be proactive about your mental, emotional, and physical health is not selfish or self-centered; in fact, it's the opposite. When you make the time to take care of yourself, the people around you get the pleasure of being around the best you possible.

Never feel guilty for taking the time to pamper yourself. Whether it is setting aside an hour a day to soak in a tub with essential oil–infused bath salts or reading a book while diffusing lavender essential oil, a daily self-care ritual is a highly valuable investment of your time.

Now that you know how you can invest in yourself using aromatherapy, chapter 3 explains how you can experience the benefits of aromatherapy by using essential oils safely and mindfully.

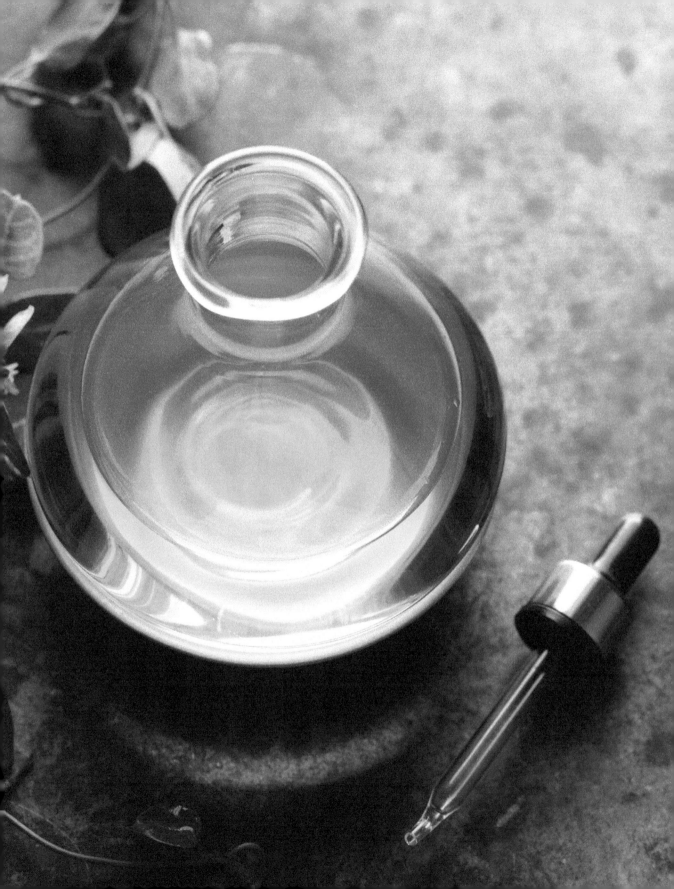

3

ESSENTIAL SAFETY

Healing with essential oils begins with safety. Learning how to properly use these highly potent oils is imperative in order to take full advantage of the therapeutic benefits they offer. This chapter includes safety information such as dosages, proper dilution, and who should (or should not) use essential oils and aromatherapy.

Risks of Improper Use

With a rise in the popularity of essential oils, there has also been a rise in adverse reactions to oils. Most documented cases of adverse reactions happened because users did not follow proper safety protocols. Applying essential oils incorrectly or using the wrong oils can cause allergic reactions (sometimes severe), skin irritation, severe pain, and respiratory failure. Treat essential oils like you would prescription medications: Use as directed and with caution.

Cautionary Oils

Some essential oils carry more risks than others. For example, some essential oils are considered "hot," which means that when applied to the skin, they carry a greater risk of causing rashes, burns, or other irritations. You may notice a slight burning sensation when you apply hot oils to the skin. Hot oils include oregano, thyme, cinnamon bark, cassia, clove, hyssop, ocotea, black pepper, and even lemongrass. Lemongrass may not feel like a hot oil to some, but each person reacts differently. Always err on the side of caution when using these oils and follow proper dilution guidelines.

Another category of cautionary oils is phototoxic oils. These may cause skin issues if they are applied prior to sun exposure. Most phototoxic oils are citrus oils, which contain organic chemical compounds called furanocoumarins that react in the presence of UV exposure. The reaction could last for several weeks and include blistering, swelling, and a noticeable darkening or reddening of the skin where the oils were applied. Phototoxic essential oils include bergamot, grapefruit, cold-pressed lime, cold-pressed lemon, mandarin leaf, rue, bitter orange, and angelica root.

Oils that contain the constituent thujone may have neurotoxic effects and should be avoided unless otherwise instructed by a trained professional. These include wormwood, mugwort, and tansy. Pennyroyal essential oil should NEVER be used. It contains pulgeone, a toxic substance that is harmful in even small amounts.

Some oils may cause seizures in those with seizure disorders. These include sweet birch, ho leaf, lavender (Spanish and spike), rosemary, pennyroyal, hyssop, sage (Dalmatian and Spanish), tansy, western red cedar, thuja, wintergreen, and yarrow.

Some essential oils have potentially carcinogenic constituents and should be avoided. These include bitter almond, fig leaf, cade, mustard, camphor, boldo, pine (Huon), horseradish, black tea tree, wormseed, snakeroot, savin, and sassafras.

Ingesting

This book will not ask readers to ingest essential oils, as this practice is generally unsafe. Many trained aromatherapists will agree that there are other application methods work just as well and are much safer. Because essential oils are the potent product of a great amount of plant material, it is potentially dangerous to ingest them due to the concentrated amounts of constituents being introduced to the liver and kidneys. Furthermore, adding oils to water can cause burns in the esophagus and mouth. The oil and water do not mix properly, leaving high amounts of the oils to come into contact with body tissues.

Pulling

Oil pulling is the practice of swishing oils in the mouth for a specified amount of time and then spitting them out. The goal is to remove toxins from the body and mouth. However, there are some drawbacks to oil pulling, especially when essential oils are added to the mix. The potential to accidentally ingest the oils or cause irritation in the mouth is real, and for this reason, this book will not ask readers to try oil pulling.

Pregnancy

Exercise extra caution when using essential oils during pregnancy or while breast-feeding. During pregnancy, the body is changing and hormones are fluctuating, which can increase the potential for issues. Additionally, some oils have constituents that may cause miscarriage or pose a risk to the fetus.

According to the Using Essential Oils Safely website, oils to avoid in pregnancy and breastfeeding include anise, star anise, araucaria, Artemisia, Atractylis, sweet birch, black seed, buchu, lesser calamint, cassia, chaste tree, cinnamon bark, costus, blue cypress, Indian dill seed, fennel (bitter and sweet), feverfew, genipi, hibawood, ho leaf, hyssop, lanyana, Spanish lavender, mugwort (common and great), myrrh, aniseed myrtle, oregano, parsley leaf, parsley seed, pennyroyal, rue, sage (Dalmatian and Spanish), savin, tarragon, thuja, western red cedar, wintergreen, wormwood, sea wormwood, white wormwood, and green yarrow.

Using peppermint essential oil while breastfeeding is fine for some, but some have experienced a reduction in milk production after using this oil.

Whenever possible, use safe essential oils via inhalation instead of topically during pregnancy.

HEALING FOR TWO

During pregnancy, essential oils can help reduce stress and promote relaxation, especially when dealing with exhaustion and frazzled nerves. How one feels while pregnant can affect the fetus. Do your best to manage any stress or anxiety with the help of aromatherapy. Not only will essential oils like lavender, chamomile, and geranium help give you a sense of calm and tranquility, but they can also help you get the rest you need to be healthy. A parent mom makes a healthy baby!

Other essential oils that are considered safe for pregnancy include bergamot, cedarwood, cinnamon leaf, citronella, cypress, eucalyptus, frankincense (carterii, sacra, frereana, and serrata), ginger, helichrysum, jasmine, lavender (Bulgarian and French), lemon, lime, mandarin, neroli, orange, patchouli, black pepper, petitgrain, pine, rose, rosemary, sandalwood, spearmint, tangerine, tea tree, valerian, vanilla, vetiver, and ylang-ylang.

Always do your research before using an essential oil while pregnant, and make sure you are consulting credible sources, not a company or company representative trying to sell their oils.

Seniors

Aromatherapy can have a wide array of potential benefits for seniors when used properly. It's important to watch for medication interactions with certain essential oils. Some essential oils can interact with specific medications and pose a risk. Always check with your doctor before using an essential oil if you are on medication of any kind. For example, essential oils like cinnamon, clove, basil, oregano, and thyme can inhibit blood clotting and should not be used while you are taking blood thinners of any kind. Oils that may inhibit blood clotting should not be used two weeks before or after any surgery, or by anyone with hemophilia. Talk to your health care provider, as well as a trained aromatherapist, before using any essential oil while taking any medication.

Children

There are times when it may be useful to try aromatherapy with children. However, it is best to wait until a child is at least two years old before using any essential oil topically. It is always best to try inhalation or diffusion first. Even then, there are some oils to avoid using for children. Eucalyptus and rosemary essential oils should be not be used around children under the age of 10. These oils can cause respiratory distress because of the constituent 1,8 cineole. Peppermint does not contain as much 1,8 cineole as other oils, so it can be used on children over the age of six. Do not use hot oils like oregano, cinnamon, and thyme around children. Oregano essential oil is not the same as oil of oregano. Oil of oregano is a carrier oil that has been infused with the oregano herb. This is safe to use with children. NEVER put essential oils in a child's (or adult's) ear. Be cautious when using premade blends with children, and research each ingredient before use. Whenever possible, try other natural remedies, such as herbs, before using essential oils with children.

Babies

Generally, it is best to avoid using essential oils around babies. This is because a baby's immune system is still forming, a baby's skin is thin, and the risk for a reaction is high. After six months of age, some child-safe essential oils may be used (if other resources have been exhausted). Although using essential oils with young children is not advised, if oils must be used, it should be via diffusion. Always make sure the oil is safe for use around children (i.e., it is not a "hot" oil or an oil containing 1,8 cineole). Second, make sure to only use one oil at a time and not multiple oils or blends. This is important in case there is a reaction: If you are using multiple oils, you won't know which one caused the reaction. When diffusing, only diffuse for up to 10 minutes and then turn off the diffuser. You can repeat this after an hour or so, if desired.

Pets

Avoid using essential oils on or around your pets. Cats and dogs respond to essential oils differently than we do. What seems safe and harmless for us may be toxic to them. Cats are much more sensitive to essential oils and should not be exposed to them.

Never Use Neat Oils

Never use any essential oil before properly diluting it. Using essential oils undiluted is called using them "neat." This practice is highly inadvisable for several reasons. First, the chances of a skin reaction or allergic reaction are much higher when using oils neat. Second, diluting an essential oil in a carrier oil actually helps the essential oil increase its surface area on the skin and enhances its therapeutic effects. If you have ever been told that an oil is safe to use neat because the company selling it only makes "pure" oils, consider this a red flag. Just because something comes from nature and is "pure" does not mean it is harmless. Arsenic and cyanide are "pure and natural" substances found in nature that are extremely poisonous.

Dilutions

Dilution is an important part of aromatherapy. Proper dilution varies depending on the oil and factors such as age, pregnancy, overall health, medications, and skin sensitivity. Generally, from ages two to six years, a 0.25 percent dilution is best. From ages six to adulthood, a 1 percent dilution is advised. For healthy adults, a dilution of 2 percent is the best starting point. When you are experiencing a health issue and want to use essential oils for healing, you may increase that dilution to anywhere from 3 to 10 percent.

For a baseline, a 1 percent dilution is one drop of essential oil in a teaspoon of carrier oil, typically a vegetable oil used to dilute an essential oil that can be anything from coconut oil to olive oil. To make a dilution, it helps to have a few simple tools. Keep a supply of small bottles for making and storing your dilutions and blends. A tiny funnel that fits a small opening comes in handy for pouring the carrier oil into small bottles. Pipettes, or small plastic droppers, make it easier to measure by drops and to transfer an essential oil from one bottle to another.

For a simple example, say you wanted to create a remedy with lavender essential oil to help combat a minor burn. You start by using a pipette to extract a small amount of the essential oil and placing one drop in another clean, empty glass bottle. Next, place the funnel on the bottle and add a teaspoon of carrier oil (like olive oil). Cap the bottle tightly and shake the bottle gently to mix the diluted remedy. Dab a small amount onto the affected area. This simple remedy is considered a 1 percent dilution. If you do not see results, you can gradually increase this dilution by adding more oil (see chart on the next page).

DILUTION CHART

Dilution	Carrier oils	Essential Oils
1%	1 tsp	1 drop
2%	1 tsp	2 drops
3%	1 tsp	3 drops
4%	1 tsp	4 drops
5%	1 tsp	5 drops
6%	1 tsp	6 drops
7%	1 tsp	7 drops
8%	1 tsp	8 drops
9%	1 tsp	9 drops
10%	1 tsp	10 drops

Safe Substitutions

There may be times when you want to substitute one essential oil for another with the same or similar benefits because of safety concerns or personal preference. For example, peppermint essential oil may not be safe to use on a four-year-old child, but you might be able to use spearmint essential oil instead. Both are in the mint family and can be helpful for respiratory and digestive issues. Here are several other safe substitutions:

- For children, consider using cedarwood or pine instead of eucalyptus when addressing respiratory issues.

- Substitute tea tree for oregano oil if you have sinus issues or need an oil with antimicrobial properties. Oregano oil can be too strong for some people.

- Lavender can be an effective substitute for chamomile for those allergic to plants in the *Asteraceae* (*Compositae*) family. Both oils are known to help reduce stress and provide a sense of calm.

- During pregnancy, you can substitute patchouli for myrrh essential oil, as myrrh is not advised for use during pregnancy. Both have wonderful skin-healing and grounding properties.

- Consider substituting black pepper for wintergreen essential oil if you are concerned about interaction with blood-thinning medications or bleeding. Both can provide relief from sore muscles and muscle spasms.

Safe Dosage

Proper dosages vary and depend on a person's age and health, the oil used, and many other factors. A safe dosage will not require a person to repeatedly apply an oil throughout the day. Even with inhalation, there are time limits to follow. The remedies in this book include safe dosage guidelines. Always follow these guidelines as closely as possible when formulating remedies. If you notice any skin irritation or adverse reactions of any kind, discontinue using the remedy.

Skin Application

When applying essential oil remedies and blends topically, it is best to start off with the smallest dosage possible. Usually, this is a 1 percent dilution for healthy adults. If needed, you can gradually adjust the dosage to achieve the desired results.

Before using essential oils on the skin, always perform a patch test on a small area of skin to check for adverse reactions. Always test one oil at a time to get a good idea of what oils are safe for you. If you are prone to plant allergies, it may be best to avoid using essential oils altogether.

Never apply oils near the mucous membranes, such as the nose or eyelids, as these areas are especially sensitive and may be more prone to adverse reactions than other areas. Never apply essential oils, diluted or not, inside the ears. Those who have tried this have experienced extreme pain and discomfort as a result. Avoid getting oils in the eyes. Never apply oils topically to children under the age of two.

Inhalation

Inhalation is usually safer than topical application, but users can experience adverse reactions. Avoid inhaling essential oils if you are prone to plant allergies. Also, be aware inhalation of essential oils can affect the body internally. For example, the use of essential oils that thin the blood can still thin the blood when inhaled. Most people assume that if they are not using an oil topically, they don't have to worry, but it is always important to exercise caution and follow safe usage guidelines.

Children under six months should not inhale oils, nor have them diffused around them. When using essential oils in a diffuser, be aware of others in the room, and do not diffuse in a public space without permission. With diffusion and inhalation, follow usage guidelines and run the diffuser for a limited time to avoid sensitization.

Top 10 Tips for Practicing Safe Healing

When administering essential oils, make sure you have researched what oils should be used and how they should be used. This list comprises 10 ways you can practice safe healing when working with essential oils.

1. Always perform a patch test on the skin when using new oils.

2. Be aware of oils to use or avoid when pregnant or breastfeeding.

3. Educate yourself on safe and unsafe oils for children and babies.

4. Start with the lowest dilution.

5. Know when and when not to use phototoxic oils, hot oils, and other cautionary oils.

6. Research how essential oils may interact with your medication.

7. Avoid ingestion, which is unnecessary and can be dangerous.

8. Never use an essential oil undiluted, or "neat."

9. Be mindful of others when diffusing essential oils. This especially applies to those working in the teaching and day care professions. Unless the parents have given permission, you could be responsible for serious and adverse reactions.

10. Do not use essential oils around pets.

In the next chapter, you will learn more about the healing properties of the 20 essential oils featured in this book. We'll also look at carrier oils and their healing properties so you can understand which carrier oil to use when creating your own remedies. You'll also find a list of other helpful ingredients to work with, as well as tools that help make formulating remedies easier.

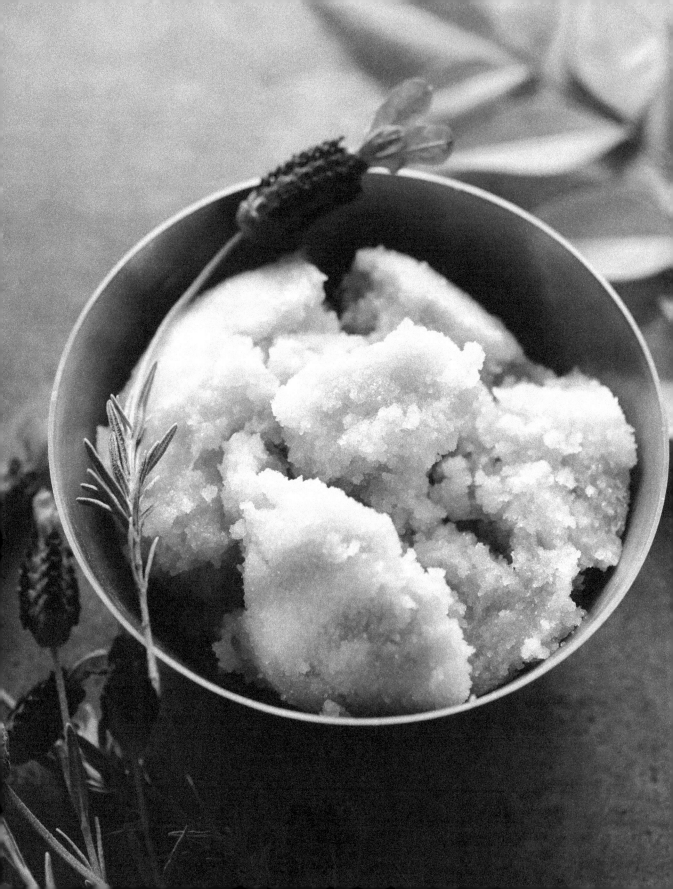

4

AROMATHERAPY FOR HEALING

In this chapter, you'll learn about specific tools
needed for healing with aromatherapy. Don't worry!
You don't need a ton of extravagant equipment to get
started with aromatherapy. You can create your own
remedies with minimal tools. This chapter describes the
items you need to have and discusses several
nice-to-have items as well.

Healing Essential Oils

I've chosen 15 key essential oils for this book based on their healing capabilities. These oils serve multiple purposes, from physical and emotional healing to beauty treatments. You'll find extended profiles for each oil in chapter 5, but here's a quick breakdown to get you started:

Clary sage: This rich, musky essential oil supports hormonal balance.

Clove: This spicy oil is a strong antimicrobial and is wonderful for combating a variety of pathogens.

Eucalyptus: With its camphorous scent, this oil can open airways fast.

Frankincense: Since ancient times, this resinous oil has provided healing due to its antioxidant content.

Geranium: With its comforting floral aroma, geranium can help calm nerves and provide nourishment to the skin.

Grapefruit: Bursting with citrusy notes, grapefruit can uplift and energize.

Lavender: Arguably the most popular oil, lavender can help combat stress as well as heal skin irritations.

Lemon: Lemon essential oil is both cleansing and uplifting.

Lemongrass: This oil can help provide a sense of peace and well-being.

Patchouli: Patchouli has a wonderfully woody aroma and is great for the skin.

Peppermint: If you are in need of invigoration and energy, peppermint can help. It also provides a lovely cooling feeling.

Roman chamomile: With both sedative and antispasmodic properties, this herbaceous-scented oil can provide relief for many ailments.

Rosemary: Rosemary is stimulating and cleansing. It can help provide relief for congestion as well.

Tea tree: Tea tree is high in antiseptic properties, making it excellent for wound and skin care.

Thyme: Thyme essential oil is a heavy hitter when it comes to killing germs.

NICE-TO-HAVE OILS

In addition to the **15** key essential oils, here are five nice-to-have oils for healing, also profiled in chapter **5**.

BERGAMOT: This citrus essential oil is famous for its mood-enhancing and uplifting properties as well as for what it can do for the skin.

CEDARWOOD: This gentle yet purifying oil is great for children and adults alike.

CINNAMON: Another spicy oil, cinnamon can kill viruses and other pathogens on contact.

GINGER: This highly anti-inflammatory essential oil has many practical uses, ranging from helping with nausea and upset stomach to fighting inflammation.

VETIVER: Vetiver is great for grounding the emotions and relieving from mental stress.

Carrier Oils

Carrier oils are an important part of healing with aromatherapy. These oils are created from the fatty part of various plants and can be used to help dilute essential oils for safe and effective topical use. Each carrier oil has its own benefits, so you can choose one based on your specific needs. Here are some popular carrier oils:

Jojoba oil: This carrier oil is smoothing and moisturizing for the skin. It is a great choice for those with sensitive skin that needs extra moisture and protection, and it absorbs into the skin nicely when applied in small amounts. Jojoba oil is also the longest-lasting carrier oil.
Con: It is actually a type of wax, so it may be too heavy for those seeking a light, greaseless oil.

Grapeseed oil: This carrier oil is a great choice for almost all skin types. It can be great for softening the skin and providing a greaseless finish. This oil is very light and absorbs into the skin well. It's also benign and can be used by those with nut allergies in place of other carrier oils.
Con: This oil may go rancid faster than others, so watch the expiration date.

Coconut oil: Coconut oil is one of the most useful and multipurpose carrier oils out there. Because of its natural antifungal properties, it is great for treating fungal issues, as well as moisturizing the skin. Coconut oil is solid at room temperature but melts to a liquid at around 78 degrees Fahrenheit; because of this unique consistency, it is a great carrier for making whipped lotions and creams.

Con: Its solid consistency can make it difficult to blend oils correctly without melting it first.

Olive oil: Olive oil may be a common staple in the kitchen, but it is also a great carrier oil for creating various essential oil remedies. It nourishes the skin and is full of beneficial anti-aging and moisturizing compounds. Olive oil can be found in virtually all grocery stores, but make sure to look for the highest quality possible. Organic extra-virgin olive oil is preferred.

Con: This oil can be a bit thick for some tastes.

Rosehip oil: This oil is a great choice for those with mature skin. It contains compounds that fight the signs of aging. The fatty acids in rosehip oil help combat inflammation of the skin, as well as wrinkles, age spots, and more.

Con: It may be a bit pricier than others.

Avocado oil: This carrier oil is highly nourishing to the skin, especially skin in need of intense moisturizing. Avocado oil is great for aging or dry skin, as well as skin affected by sun or wind exposure.

Cons: It can be very thick and often needs to be mixed with a lighter oil.

Hydrosols

Hydrosols are one of the most underrated of all essential oil-related products. This may be because many people are not sure what they are or how they are created. Hydrosols, or "floral water" as they are sometimes called, are the aqueous byproducts of the essential oil distillation process. They are heavily infused with the plant being distilled and contain small amounts of essential oil. At the end of the distillation process, the essential oils are floating on top of the hydrosol. After the oils are collected, the hydrosol is bottled for therapeutic. Hydrosols are a safe and effective remedy for those with sensitive skin, including children. Because they are water-based, they can be purchased in spray bottles for convenient use. They do not need to be diluted and can be directly applied. Below are some popular hydrosols and their uses:

Lavender hydrosol: Because lavender is strongly antimicrobial, lavender hydrosol makes a very useful remedy for spraying on minor wounds and skin irritations. It can also be used to clean surfaces prone to microbes, like yoga mats. Easy and convenient to use, lavender hydrosol provides the benefits of lavender and is safe for use on sensitive skin and around young children.

Cons: The beneficial properties of lavender hydrosol are not as strong as the essential oil. All hydrosols also have relatively short shelf lives compared to essential oils.

Peppermint hydrosol: Peppermint essential oil is problematic for some: The sensation it causes can be overstimulating for those with sensitive skin. Peppermint hydrosol is a great alternative and much safer for use on children.

Con: The hydrosol is not as strong as the essential oil, so it may not be as useful for helping with pain and related conditions.

Rose hydrosol: This hydrosol is a popular part of many natural beauty routines because the astringent and calming properties of rose can soothe and repair skin. A hydrosol is a great way to nourish the skin with a light, airy distribution that won't weigh skin down.

Con: Follow the expiration date, as hydrosols have a shelf life that is much shorter than essential oils.

Chamomile hydrosol: Chamomile hydrosol is a good choice for misting on bedding, as well as the skin, to promote calm and restfulness. There is a much lower chance of allergic reaction when using hydrosol as opposed to chamomile essential oil.

Con: Although the hydrosol is much safer than the essential oil, those who are allergic to chamomile must still exercise caution when using the hydrosol.

Helichrysum hydrosol: This hydrosol is a much more budget-friendly way to enjoy the healing benefits of helichrysum. It can provide relief from minor skin issues like inflammation, redness, and skin irritation. Helichrysum hydrosol is very effective when used on a compress.

Con: The hydrosol may not be as strong as the essential oil for treating minor sprains and inflammation.

Curating Your Apothecary

Once you determine what your healing needs are, you can decide which oils and materials to purchase. Creating your own healing apothecary can be done mindfully and in a way that aims to help you manage the everyday issues you face. For example, if you are interested in healing your skin, you may want choose a few oils that are best for the skin, as well as some carrier oils that would benefit your skin tone and health. Essential oils like geranium, frankincense, and lavender, along with carrier oils such as jojoba and rosehip, would be perfect for this. If you are interested in remedies that can nourish your mental and emotional well-being, you may want to invest in a personal inhaler or a diffuser to experience the benefits they offer. There is no need to go out and buy every single essential oil mentioned in this book if your goal is to set up a targeted apothecary. Choose your oils and materials carefully, and with a specific goal in mind.

Other Ingredients

Some remedies in this book may require additional ingredients to create an especially effective and therapeutic formulation. Ingredients like witch hazel extract, aloe vera, and unscented castile soap can further enhance the usefulness of essential oils. The following ingredients are great to have on hand while preparing some of the recipes in this book:

- *Aloe vera:* Purchasing food-grade aloe vera gel, or simply using the gel from one of your aloe plants at home, will come in handy for some remedies in this book. Aloe vera gel is soothing and anti-inflammatory, so it makes a great complement to topical remedies for pain, burning, and swelling.

- *Beeswax:* This natural substance is extremely useful for creating moisturizing and emollient salves, lip balms, or lotion bars.

- *Bentonite clay:* Bentonite clay is great for absorbing and removing impurities. It works well in remedies for detoxification and can be used in bath soaks as well as clay masks.

- *Cocoa butter:* This luscious butter is great for enhancing any lotion's skin-healing properties.

- *Distilled water:* Distilled water has a long shelf life and can be used to dilute oils for use in face and body sprays. Just make sure to shake before using a spray made with distilled water, as the oils will eventually float on top after it settles.

- *Epsom salts:* Epsom salts are a nice addition to remedies that seek to provide therapeutic support in the form of a bath. Epsom salts help the muscles relax.

- *Oatmeal:* Adding oatmeal to certain remedies can help create a soothing, anti-inflammatory skin treatment. It is a great addition to mask recipes.

- *Shea butter:* Shea butter is extracted from the nuts of the shea tree. Its moisturizing, anti-inflammatory, and antioxidant properties make it a wonderful addition to remedies targeting a wide variety of skin issues.

- *Sugar or salt:* Use either of these household staples in natural remedies that smooth and exfoliate the skin.

- *Unscented liquid castile soap:* This simple soap makes a great base for the addition of essential oils that nourish the skin and hair. Many of the unscented castile soaps on the market can be used for everything from shampoo and body wash to house-cleaning products.

- *Witch hazel extract:* This liquid is made from the bark and leaves of the witch hazel tree. Witch hazel is toning and astringent, and it complements remedies that seek to tone the skin.

SCENTS

Essential oils fall into three main categories based on scent. Understanding these classifications makes it easy to create wonderfully aromatic and unique combinations. These categories include top notes, middle notes, and base notes.

TOP NOTES hit the nose quickly but dissipate quickly. They are usually the first notes to be detected in an oil combination. Examples of top note oils are clary sage, grapefruit, peppermint, eucalyptus, and cinnamon.

MIDDLE NOTES are warm notes that may not show up right away but begin to appear after several minutes. Examples of oils with middle notes include lavender, chamomile, and rosemary.

BASE NOTES are more intense and can last quite a while. They are usually relaxing to inhale. Some essential oils that fall into this category include frankincense, clove, patchouli, and vetiver.

If you wanted, you could also separate oils into more detailed scent categories. For top notes, this might include descriptions like "citrusy" or "minty." For middle notes, this might include a description of "floral" or "herbaceous." Base note scent descriptions may include "spicy," "woodsy," or "earthy." Combining top, middle, and base notes in a blend creates a scent that not only hits the senses from the start but also lingers long after it is applied.

Essential Equipment

If you are ready to get started on your healing journey, there are just a few items you may want to have in order to create effective remedies and fully experience the therapeutic benefits oils offer. Here are a few of my essentials.

Diffuser

An ultrasonic diffuser uses water vapors to distribute essential oils throughout a room environment. It is handy if you are interested in using essential oils for air purification or emotional wellness. Diffusers come in a variety of sizes and prices. You don't have to spend a lot to get a good diffuser, and most under $30 work well for home use.

Spray Bottles

Spray bottles provide a way to diffuse oils for bodily application as well as air purification. They come in many sizes, but the best to begin with are 2-ounce and 4-ounce bottles. Make sure to only buy glass spray bottles, as essential oils can corrode plastic. Always buy tinted bottles to protect the oils inside from sunlight, which can break them down and affect their potency. If you use clear bottles, make sure to store the remedies in a dark place. Tinted glass bottles can be purchased individually, but it is often cheaper to buy them by the dozen. Make sure that the bottles you purchase have spray lids.

Inhaler

Personal inhalers provide an efficient way to experience the therapeutic benefits of essential oils. These small inhalers usually have a cotton wick inside and holes on top. To use one, simply drop the essential oils on the wick, secure it inside the inhaler, and inhale the aromas through the holes. Make sure to look for inhalers that have a cap to prevent any spillage or mess. Inhalers are great when you are on the go because you can carry them in a purse or a pocket.

Storage Bottles

One of the most convenient bottles for remedies like lotions and sugar scrubs is a simple glass canning jar. The 4-, 6-, and 8-ounce jars are good sizes to keep handy. The wider mouths of these jars make it easy to pour ingredients. Exercise caution when using glass jars in the shower or bath—if they fall off a shelf, they may break.

SPLURGE OR SAVE?

Sometimes spending a little more money is a good idea, especially when creating remedies that enhance wellness. The first step in making any purchasing decision is to decide what your needs are and whether an oil or a piece of related equipment is something you will need for your particular issues. It may be worth it to spend a little more for a particular oil if it meets a lot of your needs. Keep in mind that high-quality oils tend to cost more than low-quality oils. There are also times when it may not be helpful to spend extra money. Ask yourself if the oil you plan to purchase is one that you will be using for a variety of purposes. If the oil or equipment is not something you think you will use at least once a week, it may be best to hold off until a later date. In addition, there is no need to buy every oil and piece of equipment mentioned in this book. Understanding your personal needs and then researching oils that will help meet these needs is a great approach to setting up a sensible and functional apothecary.

5 Things to Keep in Mind to Keep Costs Down

1. Determine what issues you want to treat. Choose two or three and keep this in mind as you go through this process.

2. Read the oil profiles in chapter 5 to determine which are best for your needs. Make a list and choose several from this list to keep costs down.

3. Browse through the remedies in chapters 6 through 8 and make a list of your 10 favorites.

4. Decide what equipment to purchase based on the remedies and oils you have chosen.

5. Decide what is best for right now, and add to your collection as your budget allows. Remember, you don't have to purchase everything at once.

Chapter 5 dives into more detail about the essential oils used in this book. You will learn more about the healing properties of every essential oil, how they are best used, and important safety information for each one.

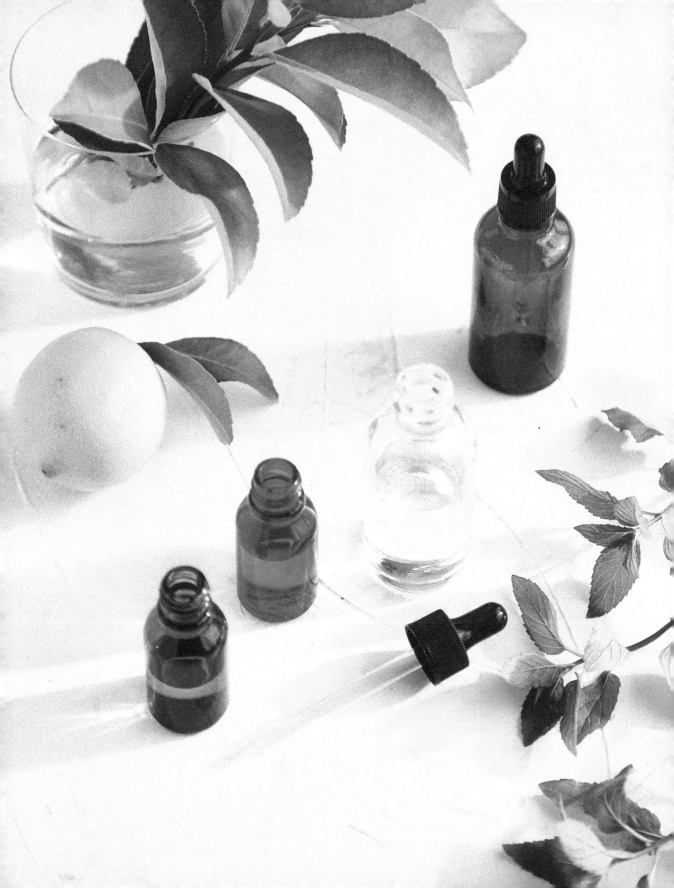

5

Key Essential Oils

There are hundreds of essential oils available on the market today. The abundance of choices can be overwhelming for someone trying to figure out what they really need for healing. The fact is, most people can get by perfectly well with a small number of versatile essential oils. The most useful and multifunctional of these oils are profiled in this chapter.

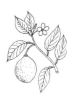

Bergamot, *Citrus bergamia*

Bergamot essential oil is usually created by cold-pressing the peels of the bergamot fruit. This is somewhat similar in aroma and flavor to an orange, but the fruit is green to yellow in color. The essential oil is lightly citrusy and uplifting. Known for its ability to bring peace and quiet to a troubled mind, bergamot has long been used for its relaxing and sedative properties. In addition, bergamot is often used in cosmetic and beauty products for its ability to tone and clear oily skin.

Healing Properties:

Antibacterial

Antidepressant

Antifungal

Anti-inflammatory

Antispasmodic

Analgesic

Carminative

Relaxant

Sedative

Toning

Ideal for Treating:

Digestive Issues

Acne and Oily Skin

Anxiety and Stress

Fatigue

Congestion

Precautions: This essential oil may be phototoxic if applied before prolonged sun exposure, so avoid use if you plan on spending time outdoors.

Substitutes: orange, lime, lemon

Uses: Because bergamot essential oil can help reduce stress and anxiety, it can be inhaled throughout the day to help manage these feelings. Its ability to calm the stomach makes it useful when massaged into the abdomen to treat indigestion. Bergamot essential oil is highly antibacterial and makes a great addition to a beauty routine for oily or acne-prone skin. The oil's uplifting aroma can also provide a sense of relaxation and optimism.

- Add one drop of bergamot essential oil to one teaspoon of carrier oil and massage into the abdomen to calm indigestion, gas, or an upset stomach.

- Add two drops to a personal inhaler to carry with you to manage anxiety and stress.

- Try bergamot in the Bye-Bye Blackheads Acne Treatment Blend recipe on page 152 for help balancing oily skin.

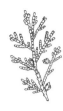

Cedarwood, *Cedrus atlantica*

Cedarwood essential oil is often created by steam-distilling the wood of the Atlas cedar tree. It has a pleasant woody aroma. Cedarwood is gentle enough to use with children yet powerful enough for adults. This rich, earthy oil can help open airways and soothes a restless spirit. Its antibacterial and antifungal properties also make it effective for a variety of skin conditions, ranging from insect bites to fungal infections. It can also help calm irritated skin.

Healing Properties:

Antifungal

Anti-infectious

Anti-inflammatory

Antiseptic

Antispasmodic

Calming

Expectorant

Insecticidal

Sedative

Toning

Ideal for Treating:

Insomnia

Anxiety and
  Restlessness

Inflamed Skin

Cough and
  Respiratory Issues

Muscle Spasms

Precautions: This essential oil is generally safe when diluted properly.

Substitutes: patchouli, fir needle, frankincense

Uses: Cedarwood helps quiet the mind and body to help you get a good night's rest. Diffusion at bedtime can be an effective way to use cedarwood for this purpose. Cedarwood can also help manage irritated, dry skin that needs nourishment. It makes a kid-friendly substitute for potentially irritating oils like peppermint and rosemary when seeking to relieve congestion. The rich, calming aroma of cedarwood essential oil is great for inhalation when you are irritated or frustrated.

- Add one drop of cedarwood essential oil to a tablespoon of carrier oil and gently massage into the face to treat irritated skin that has been damaged by the winter wind and cold.

- Diffuse three to five drops of cedarwood essential oil prior to bedtime to quiet the mind and promote restful sleep.

- Experience the healing power of cedarwood in the Tension Be Gone Bath Soak recipe on page 107.

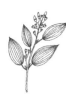

Cinnamon, *Cinnamomum verum*

Cinnamon essential oil is created by steam-distilling the bark or leaf of the cinnamon tree. The warm, spicy aroma of this essential oil can stimulate the senses and evoke feelings of tenderness, intimacy, and emotional harmony. Cinnamon is one of the most potent antibacterial, antifungal, and antiviral essential oils available. It has also been used for its ability to open airways and combat symptoms of respiratory infection.

Healing Properties:
Antibacterial
Antifungal
Anti-inflammatory
Antimicrobial
Antioxidant
Antispasmodic
Astringent
Antiviral
Calming
Circulatory

Ideal for Treating:
Viruses
Infections
Inflamed skin
Stress
Respiratory Issues

Precautions: Cinnamon essential oil can be irritating to the skin, so practice proper dilution. It may also thin the blood, so avoid if you are on blood-thinning medication. Cinnamon leaf is generally safer than cinnamon bark, which contains a compound that can be carcinogenic in high doses.

Substitutes: clove, eucalyptus, rosemary

Uses: Dr. Robert Tisserand suggests using cinnamon bark essential oil for killing airborne influenza droplets. The antiviral effects of cinnamon, when combined with other effective oils like rosemary and clove, are a powerful way to combat all kinds of viruses. Cinnamon essential oil can be used to lift the spirits and evoke feelings of warmth and tenderness. It also makes an effective remedy for congestion.

- Diffuse five drops of cinnamon bark or leaf essential oil when viruses are present in the household to combat their spread.

- Add two drops of cinnamon leaf essential oil to an inhaler when experiencing fear or anxiety to help center the mind.

- Try the Flu Fighters Diffusion Blend recipe on page 142 for help with pesky viruses, as well as relief from congestion.

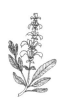

Clary Sage, *Salvia sclarea*

Clary sage essential oil is often created via the steam distillation of the aerial parts of the clary sage plant. This herbaceous and floral essential oil is a woman's best friend: It has been used for years to help regulate hormones and menstruation. This powerful essential oil can also provide serious help for symptoms of PMS. Clary sage essential oil is known for its sedative and antispasmodic properties, making it ideal for treating frazzled nerves and muscular tension.

Healing Properties:

Anticonvulsive

Antifungal

Anti-inflammatory

Antiseptic

Aphrodisiac

Astringent

Calming

Carminative

Regulatory
   (Menstruation)

Sedative

Ideal for Treating:

PMS

Menstrual Cramps

Digestive Issues

Anxiety, Nervousness,
   and Tension

Irritated Skin

Precautions: This oil may affect hormones, so exercise caution if using around children under the age of 10. When combined with alcohol, this oil may exaggerate or accelerate drunkenness.

Substitutes: chamomile, lavender, vetiver

Uses: Clary sage essential oil can be used to treat a variety of symptoms pertaining to menstrual health. It can be an effective treatment for menstrual cramps because it can help calm uterine spasms. Its ability to calm tension and frazzled nerves makes it ideal for the treatment of PMS-related anxiety and stress. Clary sage essential oil can also be soothing for the skin. It has been used in beauty products for calming skin, reducing redness, and providing relief from dryness.

- Add 10 to 15 drops of clary sage essential oil to two tablespoons of carrier oil and mix it with Epsom salts for a relaxing PMS bath soak.

- Add two drops of clary sage essential oil to one teaspoon of carrier oil and massage into the lower abdomen to combat menstrual cramps.

- Use clary sage in your skin care routine. Try the Calm and Balance Skin Toning Spray recipe on page 181.

Clove, *Syzygium aromaticum*

Clove bud essential oil is made by steam-distilling the flowers of the clove tree. The result is a wonderfully aromatic essential oil with a rich, spicy aroma. Cloves have been used since ancient times for pain relief and dental health, so it is no surprise that clove essential oil can be effective at relieving pain. In addition to its analgesic properties, clove essential oil is highly antiviral and antibacterial, making it a wonderful addition to remedies that combat colds and influenza. You can also use clove essential oil to treat fungal issues.

Healing Properties:
Analgesic
Antibacterial
Antifungal
Anti-inflammatory
Antiseptic
Antiviral
Circulatory
Immunostimulant
Nervine
Relaxant

Ideal for Treating:
Viruses
Pain
Infections
Fungal Infections
Stress

Precautions: Clove essential oil is a "hot" oil, so use topically with caution and never apply neat. Like cinnamon, clove essential oil may thin the blood, so avoid if you are on blood thinners.

Substitutes: cinnamon, rosemary, eucalyptus

Uses: Clove essential oil can be used to kill influenza pathogens, as well as those responsible for other viruses. It can provide the immune system with support to fight infections as well. Its rich, spicy aroma can help calm the senses and promote feelings of relaxation. Clove essential oil is known for its ability to help with pain and can be applied to unbroken skin (like bruises) to soothe pain and promote circulation—just make sure to dilute properly.

- Diffuse four drops of clove essential oil to help combat airborne viruses in the household.

- Add one drop of clove essential oil to one tablespoon of carrier oil and gently massage into bruised skin for pain relief and healing.

- Take advantage of clove in the Immune Booster Diffusion Blend recipe on page 144 to give your immune system the support it needs during sickness.

Eucalyptus, *Eucalyptus globulus*

Eucalyptus essential oil is often created by steam-distilling the leaves of the eucalyptus tree. The result is a powerful, invigorating scent that can open airways and promote better respiration. Eucalyptus essential oil is known for its ability to help with sinus issues, headaches, inflammation, and pain. The essential oil has a somewhat medicinal aroma, and its antiseptic properties make it effective for a variety of issues.

Healing Properties:

Analgesic
Anti-allergenic
Antibacterial
Antifungal
Anti-inflammatory
Antiseptic
Antispasmodic
Circulatory
Decongestant
Germicidal

Ideal for Treating:

Sinus Issues
Congestion and Cough
Joint and Muscle Pain
Colds
Allergies

Precautions: Eucalyptus essential oil contains 1,8 cineole and should not be used around children under the age of 10. It should be diluted properly before application to the skin, as it can cause sensitization.

Substitutes: tea tree, peppermint, rosemary

Uses: Eucalyptus essential oil is perfect for treating sinus infections because it can help open up airways and kill bacteria in the sinuses. It can also help with congestion and respiratory issues, making it ideal for diffusing when you have a cold or virus. Its analgesic properties make it similar to peppermint or wintergreen for use in a muscle rub for sore joints.

- Try a eucalyptus steam treatment for sinus issues: Boil 3 to 4 cups of water and carefully pour the water into a bowl. Add two to three drops of eucalyptus essential oil and inhale the steam coming off the water. Put a towel over your head to help catch the steam.

- Add three drops of eucalyptus essential oil to a diffuser for relief from respiratory issues.

- Try eucalyptus in the Quell the Cough Chest Massage Blend recipe on page 115 to take advantage of its antispasmodic properties when you have a stubborn cough.

Frankincense, *Boswellia carterii*

Frankincense may be one of the most popular essential oils due to this medicinal resin's use throughout ancient history. To make frankincense essential oil, one must first collect resin from the Boswellia tree. The resin is then steam-distilled to create a rich, woody essential oil. Frankincense is full of powerful properties and has been used for everything from reducing scars to easing anxiety. This powerfully antioxidant oil can even treat a variety of physical issues ranging from inflammation to digestive issues.

Healing Properties:

Analgesic

Antidepressant

Anti-inflammatory

Antimicrobial

Antioxidant

Antiseptic

Antiviral

Calming

Circulatory

Decongestant

Ideal for Treating:

Scarring

Age Spots

Inflammation

Mild to Moderate
    Depression

Congestion

Precautions: This oil is generally thought to be safe when diluted and used properly.

Substitutes: cedarwood, patchouli, myrrh

Uses: This versatile essential oil is great for helping with so many issues, from skin care to emotional well-being. It has been used to treat skin issues like acne, scarring, wounds, discoloration, and eczema. For emotional and mental issues, frankincense can help calm the mind and reduce anxiety. Its rich aroma is a powerful stress reducer. Frankincense essential oil is also effective in the treatment of physical issues like inflammation and congestion.

- Add two drops of frankincense essential oil to your favorite anti-aging serum to enhance its antioxidant and wrinkle-fighting abilities.

- Apply diluted frankincense essential oil to scars twice daily to reduce their appearance. This works especially well for keloid scarring.

- Try frankincense in the Open Up Diffusion Blend on page 96 to experience the healing properties of this versatile oil.

Geranium, *Pelargonium asperum*

Geranium essential oil presents a strong, herbaceous fragrance. It is made by steam-distilling the leaves of the geranium plant. This oil is known to be strong yet gentle enough for use on most skin types. While it has been used historically for a variety of skin issues, geranium is also great for promoting mental and emotional health, as it can help ease tension and promote relaxation. This balancing oil can help ground and center a person both physically and emotionally.

Healing Properties:
Analgesic
Antibacterial
Antidepressant
Antifungal
Anti-inflammatory
Antioxidant
Astringent
Calming
Digestive
Sedative

Ideal for Treating:
Anxiety and Stress
Digestive Issues
Fungal Infections
Wounds
Wrinkles

Precautions: Dilute this oil properly to avoid skin sensitization. It may also interfere with certain medications.

Substitutes: rose, lavender, clary sage

Uses: This useful essential oil can help treat issues of the skin ranging from athlete's foot and psoriasis to scars and aging skin. It has also been used to improve digestion. Geranium is nourishing to the emotions as well, making it useful to help alleviate mild to moderate depression, as well as nerve issues, tension, and stress. Its astringent properties help tighten and tone skin.

- Add a drop of geranium essential oil to a teaspoon of rosehip oil for a powerful anti-aging and toning facial serum.

- Add a drop of geranium essential oil to a teaspoon of coconut oil (or the carrier oil of your choice) and massage into the abdomen to combat sluggish digestion.

- Enjoy the skin-loving benefits of geranium in the Luminous Skin Hydrating Serum recipe on page 182.

Ginger, *Zingiber officinale*

Gingerroot is a very popular spice in the Far East, and in addition to centuries of use in food, it has a long history of medicinal use. The stimulating and fresh aroma of ginger is unique and memorable. Ginger essential oil is created via steam distillation or supercritical CO_2 extraction of the thick, rhizomatous gingerroot. This beneficial oil can be used for everything from treating digestive issues to combating inflammation.

Healing Properties:
Anti-inflammatory
Anti-nausea
Antioxidant
Antiseptic
Carminative
Digestive
Energizing
Expectorant
Soothing
Warming

Ideal for Treating:
Motion Sickness,
    Morning Sickness,
    or Nausea
Digestive Issues
Cough
Joint and Muscle Pain
Fatigue

Precautions: As with all essential oils, ginger should be diluted before application to the skin to avoid sensitization.

Substitutes: turmeric, peppermint, lemon

Uses: This warm, spicy essential oil can be used for digestive issues such as gas, bloating, indigestion, nausea, and constipation. Because of its anti-inflammatory properties, it can also be effective at treating pain and inflammation in the body, such as arthritis and sore muscles. It is useful at treating a variety of respiratory issues like coughs, congestion, and bronchitis. The energizing and invigorating scent of this essential oil can help uplift a tired body and mind, as well as provide energy during times of fatigue and sluggishness.

- If you need quick relief from nausea, grab a bottle of ginger essential oil and inhale deeply for several seconds. Take a few minutes' break and inhale again as needed.

- Add a drop or two of ginger essential oil to a teaspoon of carrier oil and massage into the stomach for relief from digestive issues like indigestion and bloating.

- Try the Gas Relief Massage Blend recipe with ginger on page 138 to help reduce the discomfort associated with gas and pressure.

Grapefruit, *Citrus paradisi*

Grapefruit essential oil brings on a tropical state of mind. The fresh, invigorating citrusy scent of grapefruit essential oil is created by cold-pressing the peels of the grapefruit. This is one of the strongest and most powerful citrus essential oils. Grapefruit essential oil is antioxidant-rich and beneficial for mood elevation, blood pressure, and even weight loss.

Healing Properties:

Antibacterial

Antidepressant

Anti-infectious

Antioxidant

Antiviral

Energizing

Immunostimulant

Mood boosting

Odor neutralizing

Stimulant

Ideal for Treating:

Grief

Mild to Moderate
   Depression

Viruses

Fatigue

Bacterial Infections

Precautions: Grapefruit essential oil can be phototoxic, so avoid using it before prolonged sun exposure. It can cause skin sensitization if not properly diluted.

Substitutes: lemon, lime, orange

Uses: Grapefruit essential oil can uplift and boost the mood to promote feelings of well-being and positivity, so it can be an effective treatment for sadness, depression, and grief. Its antibacterial properties make it useful for bacterial infections of the respiratory tract, and when inhaled, the oil's therapeutic constituents may work to fight infections and open airways. Its antiviral properties make it perfect for diffusion during times of sickness to kill airborne pathogens.

- Diffuse two to three drops of grapefruit and eucalyptus essential oils when you are under the weather to help open the airways and fight viruses.

- Add a drop or two of grapefruit essential oil to a personal inhaler and inhale throughout the day when you are feeling negative or down.

- Try the Get Out of Your Rut Diffusion Blend recipe with grapefruit on page 88 to help stimulate and invigorate the senses and create room for inspiration.

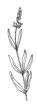

Lavender, *Lavandula angustifolia*

Famous for its calming and sedative properties, lavender essential oil is one of the most popular essentials on the market. This powerful and highly versatile oil has been proven to help reduce stress, kill bacteria, nourish skin, and heal wounds. Lavender essential oil is usually created by steam-distilling the flowering tops of the lavender plant. The herbaceous, floral scent of this essential oil makes it famous.

Healing Properties:

Analgesic
Antibacterial
Anti-inflammatory
Antimicrobial
Antiseptic
Calming
Moisturizing
Nervine
Sedative
Soothing

Ideal for Treating:

Wounds
Dry, Irritated, or
**   Red Skin**
Anxiety and Stress
Insomnia
Skin Infections

Precautions: When diluted properly, lavender is considered safe.

Substitutes: geranium, clary sage, chamomile

Uses: When it comes to covering a lot of therapeutic bases, lavender is the oil you'll want to turn to. Lavender essential oil is one of the gentlest, yet most powerful, oils available. Safe enough for use on children and adults alike, this wonderful essential oil can be used to help promote a good night's sleep, calm a restless mind, or reduce stress levels. It can be a beneficial addition to any beauty routine, as it helps soothe and calm skin in need of nourishment and moisture. This antiseptic essential oil is also great for healing wounds, burns, bites, and stings.

- Add 10 to 15 drops of lavender essential oil to a carrier oil and mix with Epsom salts for a bath soak blend that can help knock out stress and anxiety.

- Add a drop or two of lavender oil to a teaspoon of jojoba or avocado oil for a facial serum to treat dry skin.

- Use lavender for its pain-relieving properties with the Migraine Defense Inhalation Blend recipe on page 128.

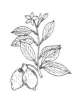

Lemon, *Citrus limon*

Lemon essential oil has a wonderfully vibrant aroma full of citrusy notes. It is known for its ability to cleanse and disinfect, as well as help with respiratory issues and boost the immune system. Like most citrus essential oils, lemon essential oil is usually created by cold-pressing the peels of the lemon. The result is a dazzlingly effervescent oil that packs a powerful therapeutic punch.

Healing Properties:

Antibacterial

Antiviral

Cleansing

Decongestant

Immunostimulant

Invigorating

Mood boosting

Stress reducing

Refreshing

Toning

Ideal for Treating:

Acne and Oily Skin

Viruses

Respiratory Issues

Age Spots

Mild to Moderate
   Depression

Precautions: Do not use lemon essential oil before sun exposure, as it can be phototoxic. Always dilute to avoid skin sensitization, as this oil can irritate sensitive skin in heavy doses.

Substitutes: grapefruit, lemongrass, bergamot

Uses: Lemon essential oil can be used to manage acne-prone skin and control the sebum that causes acne. Its antibacterial properties make it great for killing bacteria that lead to acne. Lemon essential oil can also help reduce the appearance of age spots and discoloration, making skin appear more luminous and even-toned. This essential oil has been shown to improve a dull mood with its invigorating and uplifting aroma. It has been used to stimulate the immune system, fight viruses, and aid in respiration for those suffering from colds and related conditions.

- Diffuse three to five drops of lemon essential oil when you have a cold to open airways, kill bacteria, and replenish depleted energy.

- If you are feeling down, try adding a drop of lemon essential oil to a personal inhaler and enjoying for several minutes to boost the spirits.

- Try the Luminous Skin Hydrating Serum recipe on page 182 to take advantage of the skin-boosting properties of lemon essential oil.

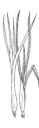

Lemongrass, *Cymbopogon flexuosus*

Lemongrass, a tall tropical grass, gets its name from its strongly scented leaves. Its aroma is very close to lemon essential oil, but with slightly herbaceous notes as well. Lemongrass has been used medicinally for thousands of years to treat a variety of conditions, and the essential oil is a powerful concentration of this aromatic plant. Lemongrass essential oil is obtained by steam-distilling the leaves of the plant.

Healing Properties:
Analgesic
Antibacterial
Antifungal
Anti-inflammatory
Antimicrobial
Antiviral
Cleansing
Digestive
Mood Boosting
Regulatory (blood pressure)

Ideal for Treating:
Fungal Infections
Sore Muscles
Digestive Issues
Viruses
High Blood Pressure

Precautions: This essential oil may interfere with certain medications. Avoid use on sensitive and damaged skin. Dilute properly to avoid sensitization, as this oil can cause skin irritation when used improperly.

Substitutes: lemon, tea tree, eucalyptus

Uses: Lemongrass essential oil's fresh, clean aroma can help boost the mood and is great for easing tension and stress at the end of a long day. It may even help lower high blood pressure. Its antibacterial properties make it an effective oil for dealing with viral issues. It has been used on the nails to treat fungal infections and works especially well for this purpose when combined with tea tree essential oil. You can massage it into the abdomen to help with digestive issues and stomach pains or discomfort.

- Add three to five drops of lemongrass essential oil to your diffuser when you feel like you need to de-stress and wind down at the end of a long day.

- Add two drops of lemongrass essential oil and two drops of tea tree oil to a teaspoon of grapeseed oil and massage into nails twice daily to treat fungal issues.

- Use lemongrass to deodorize naturally with the Invigorating Natural Deodorant Body Spray recipe on page 161.

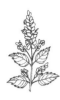

Patchouli, *Pogostemon cablin*

The rich, woody aroma of patchouli essential oil is most often created by steam-distilling the leaves of the patchouli plant. Some describe the unique scent of patchouli as earthy or wine-like. It is no mystery that patchouli boasts astonishing powers when it comes the skin and the mind alike. This full-bodied essential oil can help calm the body as well as inflamed and irritated skin.

Healing Properties:

Antidepressant

Antifungal

Anti-inflammatory

Antiseptic

Aphrodisiac

Calming

Circulatory

Febrifuge

Neuroprotective

Soothing (skin)

Ideal for Treating:

Mild to Moderate
    Depression

Inflammation

Circulation Issues

Fever

Irritated Skin

Precautious: This essential oil may thin the blood, so avoid if you are on blood-thinning medications. Do not use before and after surgery.

Substitutes: frankincense, cedarwood, myrrh

Uses: Perfect for use in beauty products, patchouli essential oil is highly beneficial for the skin. It can help soothe inflamed skin, as well as provide tone and balance. This oil is also helpful for treating mild to moderate depression and can promote feelings of mental and emotional wellness. Patchouli essential oil is grounding and centering, making it ideal for the management of stress and anxiety. It can help the body recover from illness by promoting circulation and reducing fever.

- Add a drop or two of patchouli essential oil to a teaspoon of rosehip oil to soothe irritated skin.

- Diffuse three to five drops of patchouli and frankincense essential oils to help ground and center the body and spirit.

- Nourish your hair with patchouli by trying the Natural Nourishment Conditioner recipe on page 167.

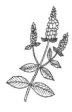

Peppermint, *Mentha piperita*

Nothing can beat the stimulating and invigorating properties of peppermint essential oil! This highly aromatic and cooling oil is famous for lowering fevers, lifting the spirits, and even providing pain relief. Peppermint essential oil is created via steam distillation of the leaves of the peppermint plant. Peppermint is also known for its ability to open airways and provide almost instant relief from headaches and migraines.

Healing Properties:
Analgesic
Antibacterial
Antispasmodic
Cooling
Digestive
Febrifuge
Invigorating
Muscle Relaxant
Respiratory
Stimulant

Ideal for Treating:
Digestive Issues
Respiratory Issues
Joint and Muscle Pain
Low Energy
Fever

Precautions: Dilute this oil properly to avoid skin irritation. It contains the constituent 1,8 cineole and should be avoided around children under the age of six. If you have especially sensitive skin, use this oil with caution, as the cooling sensation it provides can be strong. Peppermint may interfere with milk supply if you are breastfeeding. Avoid using peppermint oil if you have a G6PD deficiency or cholestasis.

Substitutes: eucalyptus, tea tree, spearmint

Uses: Like lavender, peppermint is a powerful and versatile essential oil. It is effective at reducing pain from headaches and migraines. Its camphorous and stimulating aroma makes it useful for opening the airways and promoting better breathing during times of congestion. It can be used to alleviate digestive complaints ranging from an upset stomach to nausea. Because it is so cooling on the skin, you can use it to manage fevers. It can also help fight infections and viruses.

- Inhale peppermint essential oil straight from the bottle when you need quick headache relief.

- Diffuse three to five drops of peppermint essential oil if you're congested or have sinus trouble.

- The cooling properties of peppermint make it ideal for treating hot flashes. Try the Cool It Now Spray recipe on page 131 for relief.

Roman Chamomile, *Chamaemelum nobile*

Aromatherapists often compare the smell of Roman chamomile to a crisp apple. This floral essential oil with herbaceous and apple-like notes is created by steam-distilling the flowering tops of the Roman chamomile plant. For centuries, Roman chamomile has been used for its calming and soothing properties, as well as to address a variety of other ailments.

Healing Properties:
Analgesic
Antibacterial
Antidepressant
Anti-inflammatory
Antispasmodic
Calming
Carminative
Digestive
Nervine
Sedative

Ideal for Treating:
Insomnia
Mild to Moderate Pain
Muscle Spasms
Digestive Issues
Anxiety and Stress

Precautions: Generally safe to use when diluted properly, but those sensitive to plants in *Asteraceae* should avoid it.

Substitutes: German chamomile, lavender, clary sage

Uses: When it comes to essential oils with the ability promote sleep, Roman chamomile is at the top of the list. This calming essential oil has been shown to help quiet a restless mind and body by helping the muscles relax. When combined with lavender, the effects are heightened. It can also reduce symptoms of stress, anxiety, and tension. Roman chamomile can calm a troubled digestive system and relieve stomach cramping, gas, bloating, and indigestion. It can help relieve pain when applied externally to the affected area. It makes a great addition to any skin-care routine, as it can calm red, irritated skin and restore balance. Its antispasmodic properties make it useful for muscle cramps and spasms.

- Diffuse three to four drops each of Roman chamomile and lavender essential oils an hour before bedtime if you suffer from insomnia.

- Add two drops of Roman chamomile essential oil to one teaspoon of carrier oil and massage into the abdomen to relieve an upset stomach. You can also add a drop each of peppermint and ginger essential oils to enhance the therapeutic effects.

- To use Roman chamomile for menstrual cramping, try the Don't Let It Cramp Your Style Massage Blend recipe on page 132.

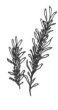

Rosemary, *Salvia rosmarinus*

The strong, fresh, herbaceous scent of rosemary essential oil is created by steam-distilling the leaves of the plant. Rosemary has been steeped in lore throughout history and thought to cure a large variety of ailments. Even Shakespeare mentioned this plant's association with memory in his play *Hamlet*. Hundreds of years later, in 2012, scientists reported that this plant does indeed impact memory, and it is being studied for the potential to help those with Alzheimer's disease and memory loss.

Healing Properties:
Analgesic
Antibacterial
Anti-inflammatory
Antifungal
Antioxidant
Antiseptic
Circulatory
Decongestant
Digestive
Neuroprotective

Ideal for Treating:
Respiratory Issues
Memory Issues
Circulation Issues
Colds and Viruses
Digestive Issues

Precautions: This oil contains 1,8 cineole and should be avoided by children under the age of 10. Dilute this essential oil properly to avoid skin sensitization, as it can be quite strong.

Substitutes: eucalyptus, tea tree, lavender

Uses: Rosemary essential oil can be inhaled to help promote healthy brain function and recall. It is great for stimulating blood flow and circulation. It can also be used on the scalp to promote hair growth by aiding in scalp circulation. Rosemary is antibacterial and a decongestant, so it's great to diffuse when you are suffering from a cold, cough, or congestion. It can help open the airways and aid respiration. Rosemary has also been used to relieve painful or sore joints and muscles.

- Diffuse two to three drops of rosemary essential oil along with a drop or two each of peppermint, eucalyptus, and clove oils to fight airborne viruses while promoting respiration.

- Add a drop or two of rosemary essential oil to a personal inhaler to carry around with you throughout the day. Inhalation of rosemary can help improve memory, in addition to soothing and calming the mind.

- Tired of short hair? Use rosemary to promote hair growth with the Tress Finesse Hair Growth Mask recipe on page 166.

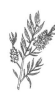

Tea Tree, *Melaleuca alternifolia*

One of the best essential oils to have in your natural first-aid kit, tea tree essential oil is a strong antiseptic and antifungal. It is created by steam-distilling the leaves of the tea tree. This herbaceous and medicinal-scented oil has a history of use for cleaning wounds to prevent infection and promote healing. This powerful oil is also popular for naturally treating acne and oily skin.

Healing Properties:
Analgesic
Antibacterial
Antifungal
Antihistamine
Antimicrobial
Antiparasitic
Antiseptic
Antiviral
Expectorant
Neurotonic

Ideal for Treating:
Allergies
Wounds
Acne
Fungal Infections
Sinus Issues

Precautions: Tea tree essential is considered safe for use but can cause skin irritation if not diluted properly. Be sure to dilute the oil generously if you have sensitive skin.

Substitutes: lavender, rosemary, eucalyptus

Uses: Tea tree oil makes a wonderful remedy for a variety of fungal infections, such as athlete's foot and ringworm. It is also an effective treatment for acne, as it can kill the bacteria responsible for creating blemishes. Use tea tree essential oil to treat minor to moderate wounds like cuts, pet scratches, and scrapes. Tea tree can help with allergies because of its antihistamine properties. Inhalation or diffusion when you are suffering from allergies can provide relief from congestion and irritation associated with allergies. Tea tree oil can help kill bacteria in the sinuses when it is diffused, making it a great remedy for sinus infections.

- Add two drops of tea tree essential oil to a teaspoon of light carrier oil, like sweet almond or grapeseed, and apply a thin layer to the face at night to help control oil and acne.

- Diffuse three to five drops each of tea tree and lavender essential oil to help control allergy symptoms.

- Try the Kid-Safe Clear the Air Blend recipe on page 143 to experience the cleansing effects of tea tree essential oil.

Thyme, *Thymus vulgaris*

Most people think of thyme as an herb to cook with, but it also has an abundance of therapeutic properties as well! The above ground parts of the herb are steam-distilled to create thyme essential oil. This wonderfully scented essential oil has an herbaceous, spicy, and sometimes strident aroma. Thyme is great for immune support and is highly antibacterial and antiviral.

Healing Properties:
Antibacterial
Antifungal
Antimicrobial
Antiseptic
Antiviral
Circulatory
Decongestant
Digestive
Expectorant
Immunostimulant

Ideal for Treating:
Viruses
Congestion
Bacterial Infections
Fungal Infections
Circulation Issues

Precautions: This is a strong oil, so it should be diluted properly before use to avoid skin irritation. Avoid use around children under the age of 10. Pregnant or breast-feeding women should consult with their health care provider before using thyme essential oil.

Substitutes: eucalyptus, rosemary, tea tree

Uses: Thyme essential oil is one of the stronger oils in terms of scent and effectiveness in fighting germs. It can be diffused to help combat the effects of viruses like colds and influenza. It can kill airborne germs, as well as those lurking on surfaces. Thyme can be diffused or inhaled to help with sinus infections and congestion. It can help open the airways and expel mucus.

- Diffuse two drops of thyme essential oil and two to three drops of tea tree essential oil to combat a sinus infection.

- Diffuse two drops of thyme essential oil and two drops each of rosemary, clove, and eucalyptus essential oils to fight airborne viruses in the home.

- Use thyme to give your immune system some help during cold and flu season by trying the Immune Booster Diffusion Blend recipe on page 144.

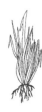

Vetiver, *Chrysopogon zizanioides*

Vetiver essential oil is created by steam-distilling the roots of the vetiver plant. This essential oil has a thick, syrupy consistency and a deep, earthy aroma. Vetiver is known for its grounding and centering effects. The scent of even a small amount of this oil can linger for hours and delight the senses. In addition to calming the mind and body, vetiver can support the immune and circulatory systems.

Healing Properties:
Antibacterial
Anti-infectious
Antimicrobial
Antiseptic
Antispasmodic
Calming
Circulatory
Grounding
Nervine
Sedative

Ideal for Treating:
Anxiety and Stress
Insomnia
Nerve Pain
Muscle Spasms
Circulation Issues

Precautions: This oil is considered safe when used properly.

Substitutes: frankincense, patchouli, cedarwood

Uses: Vetiver essential oil can be used to relieve tension in the body and mind. Its robust aroma brings balance, centeredness, and comfort to a tumultuous atmosphere. Diffusion at bedtime can promote restful sleep, especially when combined with lavender, chamomile, or cedarwood. Use vetiver for calming muscles that are prone to spasms or cramps. Vetiver can also be diluted and massaged into the skin to promote healthy circulation.

- Diffuse three drops of vetiver essential oil with two to three drops of lavender, chamomile, or cedarwood essential oil for help falling asleep.

- Add a drop or two of vetiver essential oil to a personal inhaler and inhale deeply to help you feel more grounded in the midst of confusion or turmoil.

- Use vetiver to help balance negative emotions with the Fear Be Gone Inhalation Blend recipe on page 73.

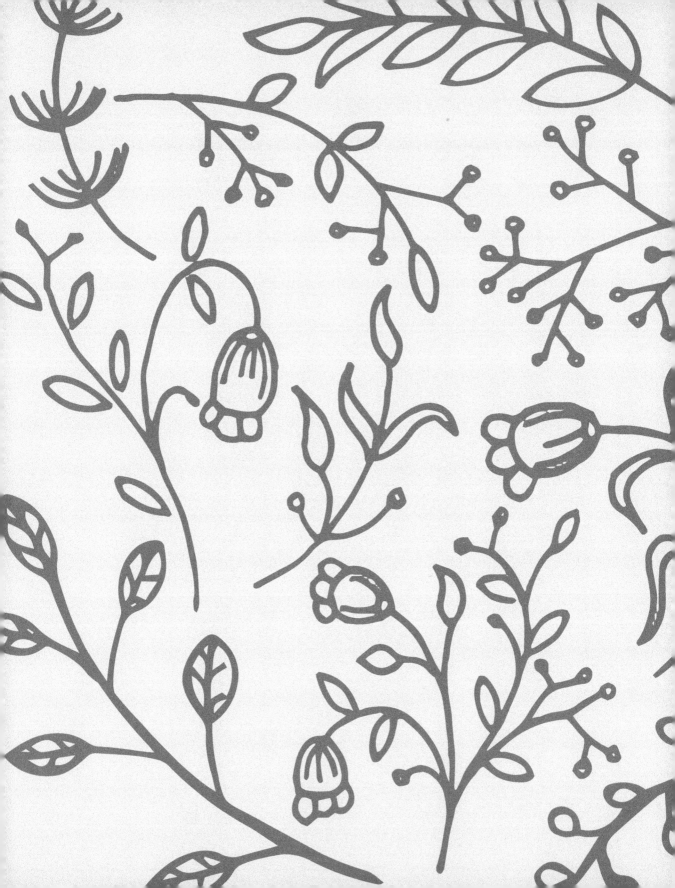

Part Two

Remedies for Healing and Prevention

The second part of this book provides detailed information on how you can employ aromatherapy to heal a variety of issues. You will find a wide array of remedies that promote emotional healing from anxiety to irritability, as well as physical healing, with remedies tackling everything from wound care to viruses. You will also find many helpful remedies you can add to your self-care and beauty routines, such as natural anti-aging skin serums and effective deodorant recipes. These remedies can help you replace many of the chemical-laden and unhealthy products you use on a daily basis with safe, natural alternatives.

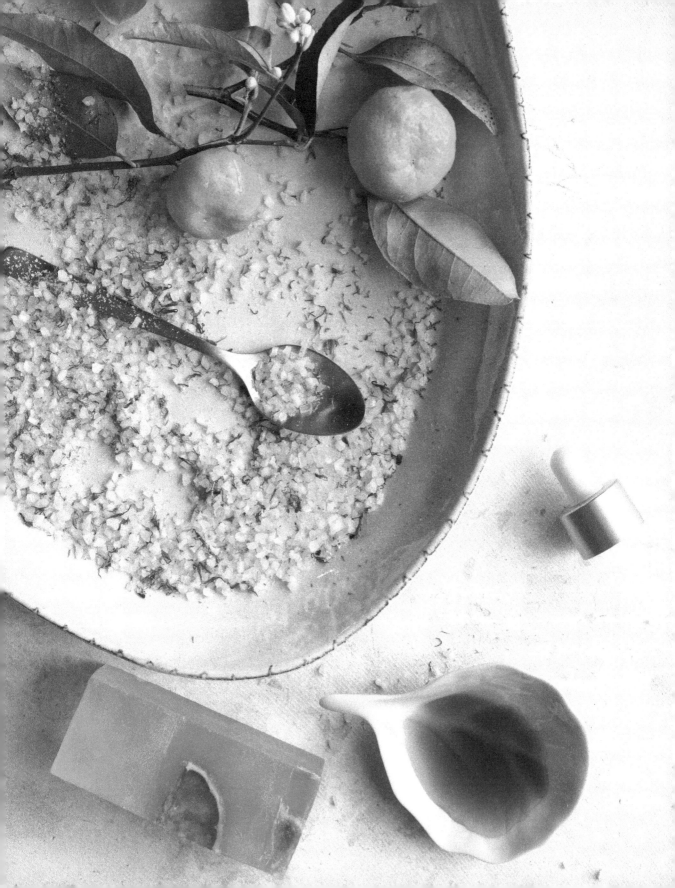

6

EMOTIONAL HEALING

The remedies in this chapter cover a variety of
common emotional ailments that aromatherapy
can help address. From anxiety to stagnation, these
ailments are listed alphabetically for your
convenience. The essential oils in each remedy
have been chosen for their particular ability
to facilitate healing.

Bye-Bye Anxiety Inhalation Blend

Scent: FRUITY AND FRESH *Makes:* 1 INHALER
Direct Inhalation: SAFE FOR AGES 5+

This blend aims to relieve anxiety and tension. Lemon helps brighten the mood and uplift, while lavender promotes calming and peace. Together, these essential oils create a wonderful scent that is sure to boost the spirits.

2 drops lemon essential oil
2 drops lavender essential oil
Aromatherapy inhaler
2 pipettes

1. Drop the essential oils into the inhaler using the pipettes.
2. Close the cap tightly on the inhaler and take three to five deep breaths of this blend when you are experiencing moments of anxiety, tension, or stress.
3. Take a five-minute break between inhalations.
4. Repeat as needed throughout the day.

STORAGE TIP: Although most inhalers have a cap, accidents can happen. To keep your inhaler fresh and avoid possible leakage, store it in a small zip-top sandwich bag.

Stay Calm Roller Blend for Panic

Scent: HERBACEOUS AND CITRUSY *Makes:* 10 MILLILITERS
Topical Application: SAFE FOR AGES 10+

In times of panic and emotional turmoil, the essential oils in this blend can help ground, calm, and soothe a troubled mind and spirit. Lemongrass is known for its ability to encourage positivity, while vetiver and lavender help with centering and calming. They make the perfect tool to have on hand for relief.

Small funnel

10-milliliter tinted glass roller bottle

9 milliliters (about 2 teaspoons) carrier oil of your choice

3 drops vetiver essential oil

3 drops lemongrass essential oil

3 drops lavender essential oil

3 pipettes

1. Place the funnel on the open roller bottle and pour in the carrier oil. Remove the funnel.

2. Drop the essential oils into the roller bottle using the pipettes.

3. Firmly place the roller top and cap back on the bottle. Shake the bottle gently to blend the oils.

4. During times of stress and panic, apply a small amount of the blend to pulse points like the wrists, inner elbows, and neck. Repeat up to three times daily, if needed.

STORAGE TIP: Keep all essential oil blends out of direct sunlight. The best place to store essential oils is in the refrigerator, as this can prolong their shelf life.

Vetiver

Frazzled Nerves Bath Soak

Scent: FLORAL, EARTHY, AND HERBACEOUS *Makes:* 1 CUP
Topical Application via Bath Soak: SAFE FOR AGES 10+

Sometimes a bath is just what you need at the end of a long day. When frazzled nerves have you on edge, combining a relaxing bath with aromatherapy can go a long way toward calming nerves and easing frustrations. This bath soak blend aims to promote tranquility.

1 tablespoon carrier oil of your choice
Medium mixing bowl
10 drops lavender essential oil
8 drops patchouli essential oil
10 drops Roman chamomile essential oil
Spoon
1 cup Epsom salts

1. Pour the carrier oil into the mixing bowl.
2. Add the essential oils to the carrier oil and blend well.
3. Add the Epsom salts and stir, making sure to evenly distribute the oils.
4. Pour the contents of the bowl into a warm bath and let the mixture dissolve. If the water is warm enough, this should take 2 to 5 minutes. Soak as long as you are enjoying the calming benefits of this blend.

TIP: For any bath soak recipe, a tablespoon of unscented castile soap will work in place of a carrier oil.

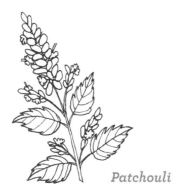

Patchouli

Regain Confidence Diffusion Blend

Scent: SPICY, EARTHY, AND FRUITY
Makes: ENOUGH FOR MULTIPLE 20-MINUTE DIFFUSIONS
Inhalation via Atmospheric Diffusion: SAFE FOR AGES 10+

This blend is for those times you feel like you need an extra nudge in order to take the next step in your life. Is something holding you back? Try diffusing this delightful blend of confidence-boosting essential oils!

Ultrasonic diffuser

3 ounces water

3 drops clove
essential oil

3 drops vetiver
essential oil

1 drop grapefruit
essential oil

1. Fill an ultrasonic diffuser with the water.

2. Add the essential oils and turn on the diffuser.

3. Let the diffuser run for 20 minutes while you practice deep breathing and meditation. Try saying positive affirmations as well. Turn off the diffuser.

4. Repeat after one hour, if needed.

FUN FACT: Research has shown that diffusing essential oils for long intervals does not provide any additional benefits; this is why many of the remedies in this book call for diffusing in short intervals up to 20 minutes. Some diffusers allow you to set intervals.

Face It with Courage Inhalation Blend

Scent: SPICY AND HERBACEOUS *Makes:* 1 INHALER
Direct Inhalation: SAFE FOR AGES 6+

Finding the courage to do what is in your heart can be difficult sometimes. This blend with uplifting and motivating essential oils can help you tackle anything that comes at you. The lavender in this blend helps bring peace and calm to get you grounded.

2 drops bergamot
   essential oil
1 drop clove
   essential oil
1 drop lavender
   essential oil
Aromatherapy inhaler
3 pipettes

1. Drop the essential oils into the inhaler using the pipettes.
2. Close the cap tightly on the inhaler and take three to five deep breaths.
3. Take a 15-minute break from inhalation.
4. Repeat as needed throughout the day.

STORAGE TIP: Although most inhalers have a cap, accidents can happen. To keep your inhaler fresh and avoid possible leakage, store it in a small zip-top sandwich bag.

Fear Be Gone Inhalation Blend

Scent: FRESH AND EARTHY *Makes:* 1 INHALER
Direct Inhalation: SAFE FOR AGES 5+

Fear can be a deceiving emotion. It holds us back from doing what is best for us and takes away our confidence. When you feel like fear is standing in your way, try this invigorating, rich, and encouraging blend.

2 drops ginger essential oil
1 drop patchouli essential oil
1 drop vetiver essential oil
Aromatherapy inhaler
3 pipettes

1. Drop the essential oils into the inhaler using the pipettes.
2. Close the cap tightly on the inhaler and take three to five deep breaths of this blend when you experience a lack of confidence or fear.
3. Take a 15-minute break from inhalation.
4. Repeat as needed throughout the day.

SWAP: If you don't have patchouli on hand, you can substitute frankincense, myrrh, sandalwood, or cedarwood instead.

Combat the Blues Diffusion Blend

Scent: CITRUSY, WOODY, AND FLORAL
Makes: ENOUGH FOR MULTIPLE 20-MINUTE DIFFUSIONS
Inhalation via Atmospheric Diffusion: SAFE FOR AGES 10+

This combination of uplifting and soothing essential oils works to bring serenity and peace. When the obstacles in front of you become overwhelming and you need to escape to a quiet place, diffusing this blend can help get you there.

Ultrasonic diffuser

3 ounces water

3 drops vetiver essential oil

3 drops lemongrass essential oil

3 drops clary sage essential oil

1. Fill an ultrasonic diffuser with the water.

2. Add the essential oils and turn on the diffuser.

3. Lie down in a comfortable spot with your eyes closed for 20 minutes. Meditate on an uplifting thought and practice deep breathing. Turn off the diffuser.

4. Repeat after one hour, if needed.

STORAGE TIP: You can run your diffuser in increments of 20 minutes (or less) until the water is gone. However, make sure you keep it in an area away from pets and children.

Pick-Me-Up Inhalation Blend

Scent: MINTY AND CITRUSY *Makes:* 1 INHALER
Direct Inhalation: SAFE FOR AGES 6+

The combination of lemon and peppermint essential oils in this blend helps stimulate your senses, uplift your mood, energize your mind, and promote a sense of emotional well-being. Inhale this blend when you feel like you need an emotional boost or are feeling emotionally or mentally drained.

2 drops peppermint essential oil
2 drops lemon essential oil
Aromatherapy inhaler
2 pipettes

1. Drop the essential oils into the inhaler using the pipettes.

2. Close the cap tightly on the inhaler and take three to five deep breaths of this blend when you are experiencing moments of mental or emotional exhaustion, or if you need an energizing and uplifting boost.

3. Take a 15-minute break from inhalation.

4. Repeat as needed throughout the day.

STORAGE TIP: Although most inhalers have a cap, accidents can happen. To keep your inhaler fresh and avoid possible leakage, store it in a small zip-top sandwich bag.

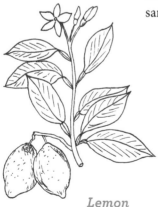

Lemon

Optimism Inhalation Blend

Scent: HERBACEOUS, WOODY, AND CITRUSY *Makes:* 1 INHALER
Direct Inhalation: SAFE FOR AGES 5+

When you feel like you need a ray of sunshine in your life, this blend is perfect. A combination of lemongrass, tea tree, and cedarwood essential oils promotes feelings of hope and light while encouraging you to see the bright side of things.

2 drops lemongrass essential oil

1 drop tea tree essential oil

1 drop cedarwood essential oil

Aromatherapy inhaler

3 pipettes

1. Drop the essential oils into the inhaler using the pipettes.

2. Close the cap tightly on the inhaler and take three to five deep breaths of this blend as needed to encourage optimism and cheer.

3. Take a 15-minute break from inhalation.

4. Repeat as needed throughout the day.

SWAP: Citronella essential oil can be used to replace lemongrass. Use only one drop of citronella essential oil in place of the lemongrass, as it can have a strong scent.

Dispel Dispiritedness Diffusion Blend

Scent: MINTY AND CITRUSY *Makes:* ENOUGH FOR MULTIPLE 20-MINUTE DIFFUSIONS
Inhalation via Atmospheric Diffusion: SAFE FOR AGES 6+

When you are emotionally drained, you may begin to feel apathetic and indifferent toward many of the things you used to love. This blend can help bring you out of this state, as well as encourage feelings of vigor, liveliness, and a zest for life!

Ultrasonic diffuser

3 ounces water

3 drops lemon essential oil

4 drops bergamot essential oil

2 drops peppermint essential oil

1. Fill an ultrasonic diffuser with the water.
2. Add the essential oils and turn on the diffuser.
3. Let the diffuser run for 20 minutes while you practice deep breathing. Turn off the diffuser.
4. Repeat after one hour, if needed.

SWAP: Orange, lime, or grapefruit essential oil can be used to replace lemon, if needed or desired. Eucalyptus essential oil is an effective substitute for peppermint, but use only one drop.

Healing from Grief Inhalation Blend

Scent: CITRUSY AND FLORAL *Makes:* 1 INHALER
Direct Inhalation: SAFE FOR AGES 5+

Aromatherapy can be a powerful tool for grounding yourself and finding positivity and healing in the midst of tragedy. This inhalation blend can promote feelings of hope, confidence, and centeredness.

1 drop lemon
   essential oil

2 drops lavender
   essential oil

2 drops bergamot
   essential oil

Aromatherapy inhaler

3 pipettes

1. Drop the essential oils into the inhaler using the pipettes.

2. Close the cap tightly on the inhaler and take three to five deep breaths of this blend as needed for feelings of grief and loss.

3. Take a 15-minute break from inhalation.

4. Repeat as needed throughout the day.

SWAP: If you are out of lemon, substitute lime, grapefruit, or orange essential oil.

Goodbye Loneliness Inhalation Blend

Scent: EARTHY *Makes:* 1 INHALER
Direct Inhalation: SAFE FOR AGES 5+

This synergy combats feelings of isolation and loneliness that so often accompany depression and sadness. Together, the oils in this blend work to provide emotional healing, hopefulness, and courage.

2 drops frankincense essential oil

1 drop cedarwood essential oil

1 drop lemongrass essential oil

Aromatherapy inhaler

3 pipettes

1. Drop the essential oils into the inhaler using the pipettes.

2. Close the cap tightly on the inhaler and take three to five deep breaths of this blend when you are feeling isolated, secluded, or lonely.

3. Take a 15-minute break from inhalation.

4. Repeat as needed throughout the day.

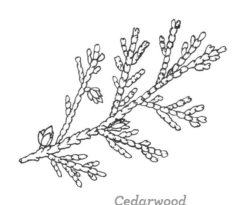

Cedarwood

Uplift Diffusion Blend

Scent: CAMPHOROUS AND CITRUSY
Makes: ENOUGH FOR MULTIPLE 20-MINUTE DIFFUSIONS
Inhalation via Atmospheric Diffusion: SAFE FOR AGES 10+

A combination of invigorating eucalyptus and citrus essential oils in this powerful blend promotes joy, exhilaration, and contentment. When you feel like you need your spirits lifted, this is the perfect tool.

Ultrasonic diffuser
3 ounces water
3 drops grapefruit essential oil
2 drops lemon essential oil
1 drop eucalyptus essential oil

1. Fill an ultrasonic diffuser with the water.
2. Add the essential oils and turn on the diffuser.
3. Let it run for 20 minutes. During this time, try to practice deep breathing techniques and meditation to ground and center yourself. Turn off the diffuser.
4. Repeat after one hour, if needed.

SWAP: If you don't have any eucalyptus essential oil, you can substitute peppermint or rosemary. Make sure no children under the age of 10 are in the room if you are diffusing rosemary, eucalyptus, or any other oil with a higher 1,8 cineole content. Peppermint is okay to diffuse around children over the age of six, but use caution.

Time to Focus Spray

Scent: WOODY AND MINTY *Makes:* 1 OUNCE
Inhalation via Atmospheric Diffusion: SAFE FOR AGES 6+

This gentle mist can be used just about anywhere to provide a comforting and stimulating effect. Essential oils like vetiver and frankincense help ground, while peppermint stimulates the senses in preparation for focus.

Small funnel
1-ounce tinted glass
   spray bottle
¼ ounce vodka
½ ounce distilled water
3 pipettes
6 drops vetiver
   essential oil
7 drops frankincense
   essential oil
4 drops peppermint
   essential oil

1. Place the small funnel on the bottle and pour in the water and vodka.
2. Use the pipettes to drop the essential oils into the bottle.
3. Firmly attach the spray cap to the bottle.
4. Shake well before each use, as the essential oils will separate from the water and float on top.
5. Make sure the spray nozzle is pointed away from your face and eyes. When you need focus, pump the spray bottle once to release a fine mist into the air in front of you.
6. Take a 15-minute break between diffusions.
7. Repeat as needed throughout the day.

STORAGE TIP: Store your essential oil spray bottles in a dark area at room temperature. Distilled water has a very long shelf life and will likely outlast the essential oils in the bottle, so expiration will depend on the shelf life of each essential oil.

Study Like a Pro Inhalation Blend

Scent: HERBACEOUS AND LEMONY *Makes:* 1 INHALER
Direct Inhalation: SAFE FOR AGES 10+

The brain-boosting oils in this blend are sure to get your neurons firing! A combination of rosemary, lemongrass, and vetiver essential oils helps stimulate and focus the mind. Use this blend when you need some serious focus.

2 drops rosemary
 essential oil
1 drop lemongrass
 essential oil
1 drop vetiver
 essential oil
Aromatherapy inhaler
3 pipettes

1. Drop the essential oils into the inhaler using the pipettes.
2. Close the cap tightly on the inhaler and take three to five deep breaths of this blend when you need help focusing.
3. Take a 15-minute break from inhalation.
4. Repeat as needed throughout the day (or night, if you're pulling an all-nighter!).

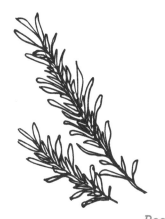

Rosemary

AROMATHERAPY AND ESSENTIAL OILS FOR HEALING

Energize the Mind Diffusion Blend

Scent: MINTY AND CAMPHOROUS
Makes: ENOUGH FOR MULTIPLE 20-MINUTE DIFFUSIONS
Inhalation via Atmospheric Diffusion: SAFE FOR AGES 10+

When our physical bodies feel drained, we can become tired and sluggish. It is also possible to become mentally drained after prolonged, extreme focus or overstimulation. This blend can help gently invigorate the mind.

Ultrasonic diffuser

3 ounces water

2 drops peppermint essential oil

2 drops eucalyptus essential oil

2 drops lemongrass essential oil

1. Find a quiet place and dim the lights.
2. Fill an ultrasonic diffuser with the water.
3. Add the essential oils and turn on the diffuser.
4. Run the diffuser for 20 minutes and try to relax and quiet your mind. Turn off the diffuser.
5. Sit still, trying not to let your mind wander, for 10 to 20 minutes.
6. Repeat after one hour, if needed.

SWAP: Rosemary essential oil can substitute for peppermint essential oil in this remedy, and tea tree essential oil can replace the eucalyptus oil.

Clear the Clouds Diffusion Blend

Scent: CAMPHOROUS AND MINTY
Makes: ENOUGH FOR MULTIPLE 20-MINUTE DIFFUSIONS
Inhalation via Atmospheric Diffusion: SAFE FOR AGES 10+

Achieve clarity with the help of peppermint, eucalyptus, and rosemary essential oils. This energizing diffusion blend can help dispel the clouds of a troubled or confused mind to bring clarity and focus. Diffuse this blend when you have trouble concentrating to help "reset" your mind.

Ultrasonic diffuser

3 ounces water

2 drops rosemary essential oil

2 drops eucalyptus essential oil

2 drops peppermint essential oil

1. Fill an ultrasonic diffuser with the water.

2. Add the essential oils and turn on the diffuser.

3. Run the diffuser for 20 minutes while practicing deep breathing techniques or meditation. Turn off the diffuser.

4. Repeat after one hour, if needed.

SWAP: Tea tree essential oil can be used instead of eucalyptus essential oil in this remedy, and spearmint essential oil can replace the peppermint oil.

Smoke-Free Smudge Spray Blend

Scent: HERBACEOUS *Makes:* 1 OUNCE
Inhalation via Atmospheric Diffusion: SAFE FOR AGES 10+

Smudging is an indigenous practice dating back thousands of years. It was done to help dispel negativity, cleanse, or bless. Resins or plants were burned to release their aromas during this practice. For those who wish to avoid burning indoors, you can create smudge blends using essential oils for a variety of purposes that help heal on many levels. This particular blend encourages grounding and centeredness.

Small funnel
1-ounce tinted glass
   spray bottle
¼ ounce vodka
½ ounce distilled water
3 pipettes
6 drops rosemary
   essential oil
5 drops lavender
   essential oil
6 drops cedarwood
   essential oil

1. Place the small funnel on the bottle and pour in the water and vodka.

2. Use the pipettes to drop the essential oils into the bottle.

3. Firmly attach the spray cap back to the bottle.

4. Shake well before each use, as the essential oils will separate from the water and float on top.

5. Make sure the spray nozzle is pointed away from your face and eyes. Spray one or two times in an open room. Wave a fan to spread the scent throughout the room.

6. Repeat every hour, as needed, for support with grounding and centeredness.

Find Your Center Bath Soak

Scent: HERBACEOUS AND EARTHY *Makes:* 1 CUP
Topical Application via Bath Soak: SAFE FOR AGES 10+

When life is chaotic and you need to get centered and find some stress relief, a bath soak with essential oils can help. A combination of clary sage and vetiver essential oils helps provide calm and grounding for the ultimate healing experience.

1 tablespoon carrier
  oil of your choice
  (or 1 tablespoon
  unscented
  castile soap)
Mixing bowl
8 drops clary sage
  essential oil
10 drops vetiver
  essential oil
Spoon
1 cup Epsom salts

1. Pour the carrier oil into the mixing bowl.
2. Add the essential oils to the carrier oil and blend well.
3. Add the Epsom salts and stir, making sure to evenly distribute the oils.
4. Pour the contents of the bowl into a warm bath and let the mixture dissolve. Soak for as long as you please.
5. Repeat daily for help with grounding and emotional balance.

SAFETY TIP: Avoid clary sage essential oil if you have been drinking alcohol, as it may exaggerate the effects.

Find Your Muse Diffusion Blend

Scent: FRUITY AND EARTHY *Makes:* ENOUGH FOR MULTIPLE 20-MINUTE DIFFUSIONS
Inhalation via Atmospheric Diffusion: SAFE FOR AGES 6+

For the times you are struggling to find the inspiration to tackle a big project, this blend can help inspire and motivate you to do your best. A rich combination of lemongrass, frankincense, and vetiver helps bring out the best in anyone seeking a deeper level of creativity.

Ultrasonic diffuser

3 ounces water

4 drops lemongrass essential oil

2 drops frankincense essential oil

3 drops vetiver essential oil

1. Fill an ultrasonic diffuser with the water.

2. Add the essential oils and turn on the diffuser.

3. Run the diffuser for 10 to 20 minutes. As you enjoy this aromatherapy treatment, attempt to clear your mind and focus on deep breathing. Turn off the diffuser.

4. Repeat after one hour, if needed.

SWAP: You may use cedarwood, patchouli, or myrrh essential oil in place of the frankincense in this remedy.

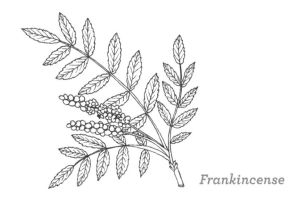

Frankincense

Get Out of Your Rut Diffusion Blend

Scent: FRESH *Makes:* ENOUGH FOR MULTIPLE 20-MINUTE DIFFUSIONS
Inhalation via Atmospheric Diffusion: SAFE FOR AGES 8+

This blend has just what you need to get going and shake off any stagnation. This stimulating combination of ginger, grapefruit, and thyme essential oils encourages motivation and vision for those seeking a powerful nudge in a brilliant direction.

Ultrasonic diffuser

3 ounces water

5 drops grapefruit essential oil

3 drops ginger essential oil

1 drop thyme essential oil

1. Fill an ultrasonic diffuser with the water.

2. Add the essential oils and turn on the diffuser.

3. Run the diffuser for 10 to 20 minutes as you relax and enjoy the uplifting fragrances. Turn off the diffuser.

4. Repeat after 30 minutes, if needed.

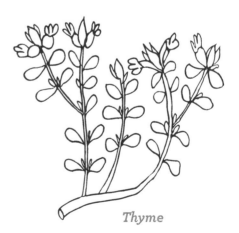

Thyme

Open Your Heart Inhalation Blend

Scent: WOODY AND CITRUSY *Makes:* 1 INHALER
Direct Inhalation: SAFE FOR AGES 5+

This gently uplifting blend increases amity and tenderness for those having trouble opening their heart. When your emotional walls are up because of past hurt or fears, this lovely blend can help take them down and pave the way for healthy relationships.

2 drops cedarwood essential oil

1 drop bergamot essential oil

Aromatherapy inhaler

2 pipettes

1. Drop the essential oils into the inhaler using the pipettes.

2. Close the cap tightly on the inhaler and take three to five deep breaths of this blend when you feel like you need emotional assistance.

3. Take a 15-minute break from inhalation.

4. Repeat as needed throughout the day

SWAP: Sandalwood or frankincense essential oil can be used in place of the cedarwood in this remedy.

Love and Tenderness Diffusion Blend

Scent: SPICY AND FLORAL *Makes:* ENOUGH FOR MULTIPLE 20-MINUTE DIFFUSIONS
Inhalation via Atmospheric Diffusion: SAFE FOR AGES 10+

A blend of warm, inviting essential oils creates a safe space for you to let your inhibitions melt away. Cinnamon, with its cheery, welcoming aroma, helps encourage feelings of warmth and tenderness. Geranium evokes feelings of being enveloped and nurtured, while bergamot promotes feelings of euphoria and encouragement.

Ultrasonic diffuser
3 ounces water
4 drops cinnamon essential oil
2 drops geranium essential oil
2 drops bergamot essential oil

1. Fill an ultrasonic diffuser with the water.
2. Add the essential oils and turn on the diffuser.
3. Run the diffuser for 20 minutes. Turn off the diffuser.
4. Repeat after 20 minutes, if desired.

SWAP: Clove essential oil can replace the cinnamon, but use two to three drops instead of four.

90 AROMATHERAPY AND ESSENTIAL OILS FOR HEALING

In the Mood for Love Massage Blend

Scent: HERBACEOUS *Makes:* 1 OUNCE
Topical Application: SAFE FOR AGES 18+

Clary sage and Roman chamomile essential oils combine in this special blend for those seeking to enhance intimacy and affection in their relationship. Both essential oils possess powerful and relaxing properties that help melt away distractions, preparing your mind and body for intimacy.

1 ounce carrier oil of your choice

1-ounce tinted glass bottle with a lid

Small funnel

6 drops clary sage essential oil

6 drops Roman chamomile essential oil

2 pipettes

1. Place the funnel on the open bottle and pour in the carrier oil. Remove the funnel.

2. Add the essential oils with the pipettes. Firmly attach the lid to the container and shake it to blend the oils together well.

3. Massage a quarter-size amount onto the back, arms, legs, and abdomen to promote feelings of openness and intimacy.

STORAGE TIP: Store this blend in a cool, dark place. Shelf life will depend on the expiration of your carrier oil, so take note of this date and label your bottle accordingly.

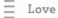

A Little Spice in Your Life Diffusion Blend

Scent: SPICY *Makes:* ENOUGH FOR MULTIPLE 20-MINUTE DIFFUSIONS
Inhalation via Atmospheric Diffusion: SAFE FOR AGES 10+

This spicy and nurturing blend can set the mood and create an enticing setting. Warm and inviting cinnamon blends with herbaceous and spicy clary sage to promote feelings of intimacy and closeness.

Ultrasonic diffuser

3 ounces water

6 drops cinnamon essential oil

4 drops clary sage essential oil

1. Fill an ultrasonic diffuser with the water.

2. Add the essential oils and turn on the diffuser.

3. Run the diffuser for 20 minutes. Turn off the diffuser.

Ramp Up Your Recall Inhalation Blend

Scent: EARTHY AND HERBACEOUS *Makes:* 1 INHALER
Direct Inhalation: SAFE FOR AGES 10+

If you're having memory trouble or feel like you're constantly forgetting stuff, this blend can help improve recall and heighten the senses. Rosemary has been shown to help with memory, and frankincense can focus the mind. Together, these oils can boost brain function.

2 drops rosemary essential oil

1 drop frankincense essential oil

Aromatherapy inhaler

2 pipettes

1. Drop the essential oils into the inhaler using the pipettes.

2. Close the cap tightly on the inhaler and take three to five deep breaths.

3. Take a 15-minute break from inhalation.

4. Repeat at least three times daily to promote enhanced brain function and improve memory.

SWAP: Myrrh or patchouli essential oil can be used in place of frankincense in this remedy.

Trauma and Trouble Tamer Inhalation Blend

Scent: FRUITY *Makes:* 1 INHALER
Direct Inhalation: SAFE FOR AGES 5+

Let the pacifying effects of Roman chamomile, bergamot, and grapefruit essential oils help you heal. This blend was formulated to aid in coping with trauma. These oils can provide a comforting and calming feeling that helps soothe troubling emotions.

2 drops Roman
chamomile
essential oil
1 drop grapefruit
essential oil
2 drops bergamot
essential oil
Aromatherapy inhaler
3 pipettes

1. Drop the essential oils into the inhaler using the pipettes.
2. Close the cap tightly on the inhaler and take three to five deep breaths of this blend when you are in need of emotional support.
3. Take a 15-minute break from inhalation.
4. Repeat as needed throughout the day.

SWAP: Orange, lime, or lemon essential oil can be used in place of grapefruit in this remedy.

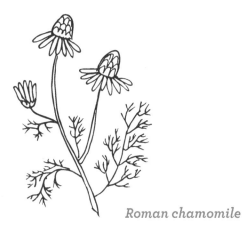

Roman chamomile

Get Rid of the Baggage Bath Soak

Scent: FLORAL AND EARTHY *Makes:* 1 CUP
Topical Application via Bath Soak: SAFE FOR AGES 8+

Soak away your troubles with this recipe for mental and emotional wellness. Patchouli and geranium combine in this bath soak blend to dispel negative emotions and promote relaxation. Use this remedy when you need to shed some unwanted baggage.

1 tablespoon carrier oil (or unscented castile soap)
Medium mixing bowl
10 drops patchouli essential oil
10 drops geranium essential oil
Spoon
1 cup Epsom salts

1. Pour the carrier oil into the mixing bowl.
2. Add the essential oils to the carrier oil and blend well.
3. Add the Epsom salts and stir, making sure to evenly distribute the oils.
4. Pour the contents of the bowl into a warm bath and let the mixture dissolve. Soak as long as you are enjoying the benefits of this blend.

SWAP: Frankincense, cedarwood, or sandalwood essential oil can substitute for patchouli in this blend.

Open Up Diffusion Blend

Scent: SPICY *Makes:* ENOUGH FOR MULTIPLE 20-MINUTE DIFFUSIONS
Inhalation via Atmospheric Diffusion: SAFE FOR AGES 10+

If you have trouble allowing yourself to share your emotions or be emotionally available to others, this blend can help you open up. Diffuse this warming combination of cinnamon, clove, and frankincense to help combat emotional unavailability or the feeling of being closed off.

Ultrasonic diffuser

3 ounces water

3 drops cinnamon
essential oil

2 drops clove
essential oil

3 drops frankincense
essential oil

1. Fill an ultrasonic diffuser with the water.

2. Add the essential oils and turn on the diffuser.

3. Run the diffuser for 20 minutes while practicing deep breathing techniques. Try reciting positive affirmations during this time as well. Turn off the diffuser.

4. Repeat daily as needed.

SWAP: You may use patchouli, cedarwood, sandalwood, or myrrh essential oil in place of frankincense in this remedy.

Anger Antidote Bath Soak

Scent: FRUITY, FLORAL, AND EARTHY *Makes:* 1 CUP
Topical Application via Bath Soak: SAFE FOR AGES 8+

If you are experiencing anger and irritability on a regular basis, it may be time to address the issue. You can start by practicing self-care with this bath soak formulated to help you shed negative emotions.

1 tablespoon carrier oil (or unscented castile soap)

Medium mixing bowl

8 drops bergamot essential oil

10 drops lavender essential oil

5 drops patchouli essential oil

Spoon

1 cup Epsom salts

1. Pour the carrier oil into the mixing bowl.

2. Add the essential oils to the carrier oil and blend well.

3. Add the Epsom salts and stir, making sure to evenly distribute the oils.

4. Pour the contents of this bowl into a warm bath and let the mixture dissolve. Soak for at least 20 minutes to take advantage of the emotional support the oils can offer.

SWAP: Geranium essential oil can be used instead of lavender in this remedy. Vetiver essential oil is a great replacement for patchouli, as it is calming and grounding.

Restlessness Reliever Inhalation Blend

Scent: FLORAL AND WOODY *Makes:* 1 INHALER
Direct Inhalation: SAFE FOR AGES 5+

Impatience can impact you in a major way if you let it. When you find that impatience is affecting your everyday life, try inhaling this blend to quiet the restlessness inside. The oils in this remedy combine to promote tranquility and centeredness so you can focus on what really matters.

2 drops lavender essential oil

2 drops cedarwood essential oil

1 drop lemongrass essential oil

Aromatherapy inhaler

3 pipettes

1. Drop the essential oils into the inhaler using the pipettes.
2. Close the cap tightly on the inhaler and take three to five deep breaths of this blend when you are experiencing moments of impatience.
3. Take a 15-minute break from inhalation.
4. Repeat as often as needed throughout the day.

SWAP: Frankincense essential oil is a great substitute for cedarwood in this remedy, as it can provide many of the same calming benefits.

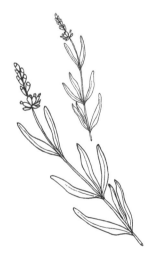

Lavender

Get Free from Frustration Diffusion Blend

Scent: CRISP AND FRUITY *Makes:* ENOUGH FOR MULTIPLE 20-MINUTE DIFFUSIONS
Inhalation via Atmospheric Diffusion: SAFE FOR AGES 5+

Everyone feels frustrated sometimes, but it becomes a problem when we let it affect our lives on a regular basis. This can lead to issues with anxiety, stress, and even our physical health. Conquer feelings of frustration with this diffusion blend.

Ultrasonic diffuser

3 ounces water

4 drops bergamot essential oil

4 drops Roman chamomile essential oil

1. Find a quiet place and dim the lights.
2. Fill an ultrasonic diffuser with the water.
3. Add the essential oils and turn on the diffuser.
4. Run the diffuser for 20 minutes and enjoy the aromatherapy session. Turn off the diffuser.
5. Repeat after one hour, if needed.

SWAP: In a pinch, lavender essential oil can substitute for Roman chamomile.

Peaceful Child Inhalation Blend

Scent: FLORAL AND EARTHY *Makes:* 1 INHALER
Direct Inhalation: SAFE FOR AGES 2+

Emotions can get the best of adults, but sometimes we forget that children have emotions too. Often these emotions can be strong and hard to control. This blend can come in handy for children who need help calming their negative emotions.

2 drops cedarwood
   essential oil

2 drops lavender
   essential oil

1 drop bergamot
   essential oil

Aromatherapy inhaler

3 pipettes

1. Drop the essential oils into the inhaler using the pipettes.

2. Close the cap tightly on the inhaler and hold the inhaler under the child's nose, encouraging them to take three to five deep breaths and enjoy the aromas.

3. Repeat after 30 minutes, if needed.

SWAP: Roman chamomile essential oil can be used in place of lavender in this blend, and frankincense, patchouli, or sandalwood essential oil can replace cedarwood.

Mood Mender Diffusion Blend

Scent: HERBACEOUS *Makes:* ENOUGH FOR MULTIPLE 20-MINUTE DIFFUSIONS
Inhalation via Diffusion: SAFE FOR AGES 10+

When PMS symptoms are giving you trouble, this blend can give you emotional and physical relief. Clary sage essential oil is famous for its mood-balancing effects, while Roman chamomile and vetiver provide emotional support. In addition, clary sage and Roman chamomile essential oils can help with uterine spasms and cramps.

Ultrasonic diffuser

3 ounces water

3 drops clary sage essential oil

2 drops Roman chamomile essential oil

2 drops vetiver essential oil

1. Find a place to relax with minimal distractions.

2. Fill an ultrasonic diffuser with the water.

3. Add the essential oils and turn on the diffuser.

4. Run the diffuser for 10 to 20 minutes and practice deep breathing techniques while enjoying the calming effects of the essential oils. Turn off the diffuser.

5. Repeat after 30 minutes to one hour, if needed.

Peaceful Pregnancy Inhalation Blend

Scent: HERBACEOUS AND MEDICINAL *Makes:* 1 INHALER
Direct Inhalation: SAFE FOR ALL AGES

Pregnancy is a time of fluctuating hormones and physical and emotional changes. Essential oils like lavender and Roman chamomile can provide support and calming during this amazing time.

2 drops lavender
   essential oil
2 drops Roman
   chamomile
   essential oil
Aromatherapy inhaler
2 pipettes

1. Drop the essential oils into the inhaler using the pipettes.
2. Close the cap tightly on the inhaler and take three to five deep breaths as needed for stress relief during pregnancy.
3. Take a 15-minute break from inhalation.
4. Repeat as often as needed throughout the day.

SWAP: Clary sage essential oil can be used in place of Roman chamomile or lavender in this remedy.

Better Birth Inhalation Blend

Scent: WOODY AND HERBACEOUS *Makes:* 1 INHALER
Direct Inhalation: SAFE FOR ALL AGES

Essential oils like lavender, bergamot, and cedarwood can nurture and comfort you during labor by lifting the spirits, relieving anxiety, relaxing the body, and inspiring feelings of optimism and joy. Don't forget to include this inhalation blend in your hospital bag or home birth kit.

**1 drop lavender
essential oil
2 drops bergamot
essential oil
1 drop cedarwood
essential oil
Aromatherapy inhaler
3 pipettes**

1. Drop the essential oils into the inhaler using the pipettes.
2. Close the cap tightly on the inhaler and take three to five deep breaths as needed for a soothing effect during labor.
3. Take a 15-minute break from inhalation.
4. Repeat as often as needed throughout the day.

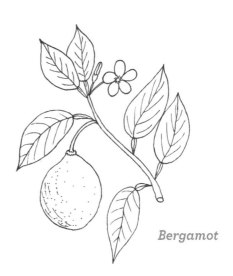

Bergamot

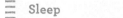

Peaceful Dreams Diffusion Blend

Scent: EARTHY AND HERBACEOUS
Makes: ENOUGH FOR MULTIPLE 20-MINUTE DIFFUSIONS
Inhalation via Atmospheric Diffusion: SAFE FOR AGES 5+

If you are one of the millions of people who find it hard to fall asleep or stay asleep at night, this blend may be just what you're looking for. The gentle combination of lavender and vetiver essential oils helps soothe the mind and body while encouraging a restful night's sleep.

Ultrasonic diffuser
3 ounces water
5 drops lavender essential oil
5 drops vetiver essential oil

1. Fill an ultrasonic diffuser with the water.
2. Add the essential oils and turn on the diffuser.
3. Run the diffuser for five to 10 minutes before going to bed. Set the time on the diffuser for 20 minutes after you turn in for the night.
4. Repeat as needed each evening to promote healthy sleep.

SWAP: Roman chamomile essential oil can be used in place of lavender in this remedy.

Sleep Well Roller Blend

Scent: EARTHY AND FLORAL *Makes:* 10 MILLILITERS
Topical Application: SAFE FOR AGES 6+

This alternative to diffusion stays with you throughout the night to bring restful sleep. The essential oils in this blend are famous for their sedative and calming effects. Together, they promote a peaceful body and mind.

Small funnel
10-milliliter tinted glass roller bottle
9 milliliters (about 2 teaspoons) carrier oil of your choice
2 drops vetiver essential oil
4 drops cedarwood essential oil
4 drops lavender essential oil
3 pipettes

1. Place the funnel on the open roller bottle and pour in the carrier oil. Remove the funnel.

2. Drop the essential oils into the roller bottle using the pipettes.

3. Firmly place the roller top and cap back on the bottle. Shake the bottle gently to blend the oils.

4. One hour before bedtime, apply a small amount of this blend to the back of the neck, on the wrists, and behind the ears. Make sure to keep physical activity to a minimum during this time and avoid screen time.

5. Use this blend nightly, as needed, for insomnia.

Escape from Exhaustion Spray

Scent: MINTY AND HERBACEOUS *Makes:* 1 OUNCE
Inhalation via Atmospheric Diffusion: SAFE FOR AGES 10+

When stress has you feeling exhausted, this blend can pick you up and provide relaxation. The combination of lavender and peppermint smells amazing as well. Because this blend is a spray, it is great for healing on the go.

Small funnel
1-ounce tinted glass
   spray bottle
¼ ounce vodka
½ ounce distilled water
2 pipettes
6 drops peppermint
   essential oil
10 drops lavender
   essential oil

1. Place the funnel on the bottle and pour in the water and vodka. Remove the funnel.

2. Use the pipettes to drop the essential oils into the bottle.

3. Firmly attach the spray cap to the bottle.

4. Shake well before each use, as the essential oils will separate from the water and float on top. Make sure the spray nozzle is pointed away from your face and eyes. Pump the spray bottle once to release a fine mist into the air in front of you.

5. Repeat after one hour, if needed.

STORAGE TIP: Store this blend in a cool, dark place. Shelf life will depend on the expiration of your essential oils, so take note of these dates and label your bottle accordingly.

Tension Be Gone Bath Soak

Scent: FRUITY AND WOODY *Makes:* 1 CUP
Topical Application via Bath Soak: SAFE FOR AGES 10+

When stress begins to cause tension, the effects can range from physical soreness to emotional frailty. This blend is perfect for those in need of a soothing, stress-relieving bath soak that aims to calm the body and the emotions.

1 tablespoon carrier oil of your choice (or unscented castile soap)
Medium mixing bowl
10 drops lavender essential oil
5 drops lemon essential oil
8 drops cedarwood essential oil
Spoon
1 cup Epsom salts

1. Pour the carrier oil into the mixing bowl.
2. Add the essential oils to the carrier oil and blend well.
3. Add the Epsom salts and stir, making sure to evenly distribute the oils.
4. Pour the contents of the bowl into a warm bath and let the mixture dissolve. Soak as long as needed. The longer you soak, the better you'll feel.

SAFETY TIP: Remember to rinse off well after your bath, as lemon essential oil can cause irritation if you go out into the sun with it on your skin.

Just Breathe Inhalation Blend

Scent: HERBACEOUS *Makes:* 1 INHALER
Direct Inhalation: SAFE FOR AGES 10+

Life is full of changes. Sometimes coping with these changes can be difficult and we have to remind ourselves to sit down and "just breathe." This grounding and uplifting blend can get you centered and ready to confront whatever you're facing. Roman chamomile essential oil brings peace, while patchouli encourages balance and grounding. Clary sage oil can help calm inner turmoil and anxiety.

1 drop clary sage essential oil

1 drop patchouli essential oil

2 drops chamomile essential oil

Aromatherapy inhaler

3 pipettes

1. Drop the essential oils into the inhaler using the pipettes.

2. Close the cap tightly on the inhaler and take three to five deep breaths of this blend when you are struggling with a transition or change in your life.

3. Take a 15-minute break from inhalation.

4. Repeat as needed throughout the day.

SWAP: Lavender essential oil is an effective substitute for chamomile, if needed.

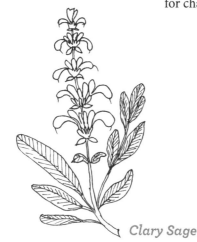

Clary Sage

New Beginning Diffusion Blend

Scent: CITRUSY *Makes:* ENOUGH FOR MULTIPLE 20-MINUTE DIFFUSIONS
Inhalation via Atmospheric Diffusion: SAFE FOR AGES 5+

When a major life transition is the catalyst for a new beginning, this blend can help encourage comfort and optimism about whatever is happening in your life. Lemon and bergamot can energize and uplift the senses, while vetiver essential oil brings perspective and support. This blend is great to use in a new home.

Ultrasonic diffuser
3 ounces water
3 drops bergamot
   essential oil
2 drops lemon
   essential oil
1 drop vetiver
   essential oil

1. Fill an ultrasonic diffuser with the water.

2. Add the essential oils and turn on the diffuser.

3. Run the diffuser for 20 minutes. Turn off the diffuser.

4. Repeat after 30 minutes to one hour, if needed.

SWAP: Orange, lime, or grapefruit essential oil will work as a substitute for lemon essential oil in this blend.

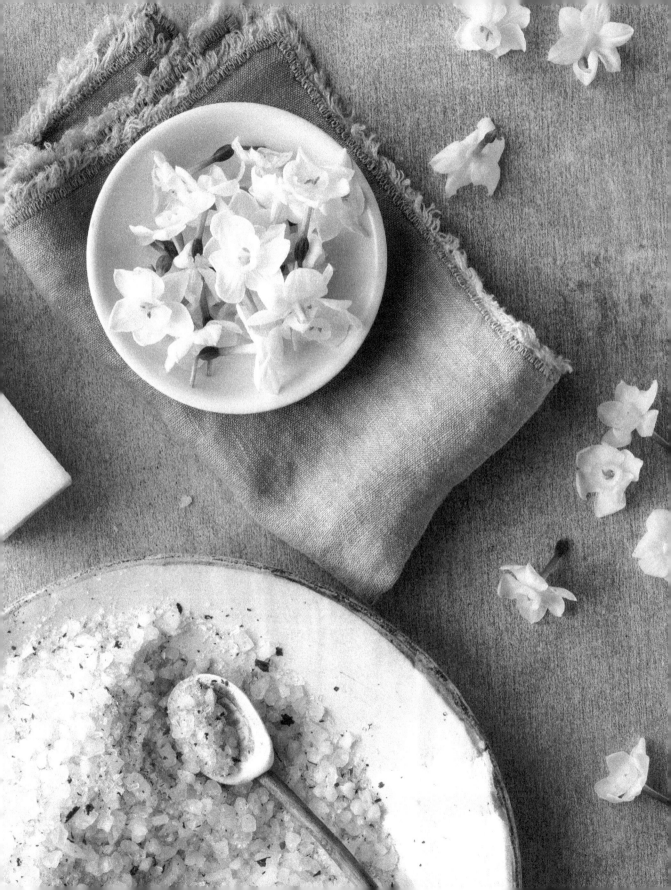

7

Physical Healing

The strength and potency of essential oils make them perfect for healing all kinds of physical ailments. Perhaps even better, the healing these oils provides has little or no side effects when used properly. In this chapter, you will learn more about what conditions can be remedied with essential oils, as well as how to create these remedies at home. Remedies are listed alphabetically by ailment.

Antihistamine Rescue Roller Blend

Scent: HERBACEOUS AND MEDICINAL *Makes:* 10 MILLILITERS
Topical Application: SAFE FOR AGES 6+

When allergies have you down, try this simple blend of tea tree and lavender essential oils. Both of these oils contain antihistamine properties, helping fight the inflammation and bodily reactions that lead to allergy symptoms.

Small funnel

10-milliliter tinted glass roller bottle

9 milliliters (about 2 teaspoons) carrier oil of your choice

5 drops tea tree essential oil

5 drops lavender essential oil

2 pipettes

1. Place the funnel on the open roller bottle and pour in the carrier oil. Remove the funnel.

2. Drop the essential oils into the roller bottle using the pipettes.

3. Firmly place the roller top and cap back on the bottle. Shake the bottle gently to blend the oils.

4. Apply to the wrists up to twice daily for allergy relief. After applying to the wrists, hold them up to your nose and breathe in the oils.

STORAGE TIP: Store all roller bottle blends in a cool, dark place out of direct sunlight. Label the bottles well, indicating the date they were created, the name of the remedy, and the expiration date on the carrier oil (this will be the expiration for your roller remedy as well).

Heal the Burn Spray

Scent: FLORAL AND EARTHY *Makes:* 1 OUNCE
Topical Application: SAFE FOR AGES 5+

This useful spray blend contains nourishing oils that can reduce the pain, skin damage, and inflammation caused by minor burns. Lavender essential oil has been shown to heal skin damage caused by burns, and when combined with antioxidant-rich frankincense, the effectiveness doubles.

Small funnel

1-ounce tinted glass spray bottle

¼ ounce aloe vera juice

½ ounce distilled water

20 drops lavender essential oil

10 drops frankincense essential oil

2 pipettes

1. Place the funnel on the bottle and pour in the water and aloe vera juice. Remove the funnel.

2. Add the essential oils using the pipettes.

3. Firmly secure the spray cap on the bottle.

4. Shake vigorously before use, as the essential oils will separate from the water and float on top. Apply to minor burns after washing the burn with cool water and drying the area well.

5. Apply as often as needed after a burn to promote healing. Do not use on severe burns or open wounds.

SWAP: Try using aloe vera juice to replace the distilled water. You can also use half distilled water and half aloe vera juice for an effective remedy.

A Breath of Fresh Air Inhalation Blend

Scent: CAMPHOROUS *Makes:* 1 INHALER
Direct Inhalation: SAFE FOR AGES 10+

When you need help opening your airways, turn to this blend of powerful oils. Tea tree, eucalyptus, and peppermint essential oils work together to promote better respiration and cleanse the sinuses. Their strong antibacterial properties are also great for fighting bacteria in the respiratory tract that could lead to infection.

1 drop tea tree essential oil
2 drops eucalyptus essential oil
1 drop peppermint essential oil
Aromatherapy inhaler
3 pipettes

1. Drop the essential oils into the inhaler using the pipettes.
2. Close the cap tightly on the inhaler and take three to five deep breaths of this blend when needed to clear congestion.
3. Take a 15-minute break from inhalation.
4. Repeat as needed throughout the day.

SWAP: Spearmint essential oil works well in place of peppermint in a pinch. Rosemary essential oil can replace tea tree oil, if you happen to be out.

Quell the Cough Chest Massage Blend

Scent: WOODY AND CAMPHOROUS *Makes:* 1 OUNCE
Topical Application: SAFE FOR AGES 10+

To combat nagging coughs and open airways, try this chest massage blend. A combination of frankincense, cedarwood, and eucalyptus oils calms irritation and breaks up mucus that leads to issues. The antispasmodic properties of the oils help prevent coughing that inhibits rest.

Small funnel

1-ounce tinted glass bottle with lid

1 ounce carrier oil of your choice

5 drops eucalyptus essential oil

6 drops cedarwood essential oil

6 drops frankincense essential oil

3 pipettes

1. Place the funnel on the open bottle and pour in the carrier oil. Remove the funnel.

2. Add the essential oils using the pipettes.

3. Close the cap tightly and shake the bottle gently to blend the oils.

4. Apply a nickel-size drop of this blend to the chest at bedtime and massage thoroughly into the skin until it is absorbed.

5. Repeat nightly until congestion and coughing have stopped.

SWAP: Cedarwood essential oil is an effective substitute for frankincense in this remedy.

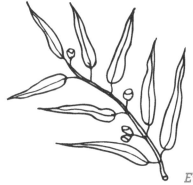

Eucalyptus

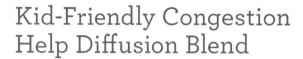

Kid-Friendly Congestion Help Diffusion Blend

Scent: WOODY AND CITRUSY *Makes:* ENOUGH FOR MULTIPLE 20-MINUTE DIFFUSIONS
Inhalation via Atmospheric Diffusion: SAFE FOR AGES 5+

Not all essential oils are safe for children, especially those that aid in respiration. This blend uses child-safe essential oils to promote opening of the airways and help with coughing and congestion that keep children awake at night.

Ultrasonic diffuser

3 ounces water

4 drops cedarwood
essential oil

3 drops lemon
essential oil

4 drops tea tree
essential oil

1. Fill an ultrasonic diffuser with the water.

2. Add the essential oils.

3. At bedtime, turn the diffuser on in the child's room. If you have a diffuser with a timer, set it to run for no more than 20 minutes. (If not, you will need to turn off the diffuser after 20 minutes.)

Healing Detox Bath Soak

Scent: HERBACEOUS *Makes:* 1½ CUPS
Topical Application via Bath Soak: SAFE FOR AGES 8+

This detox bath recipe is great when you are not feeling well, may have been exposed to toxins, or just want to relax and unwind. The bentonite clay helps pull impurities out of the body, while lavender and tea tree essential oils nourish and protect the skin.

2 tablespoons carrier oil of your choice (or unscented castile soap)
Medium mixing bowl
10 drops lavender essential oil
10 drops tea tree essential oil
Spoon
1 cup Epsom salts
½ cup bentonite clay

1. Pour the carrier oil into the mixing bowl.
2. Add the essential oils to the carrier and blend well.
3. Add the Epsom salts and stir, making sure to evenly distribute the oils.
4. Add the bentonite clay, gently stirring until the clay is blended with the salt and oils.
5. Add the mixture to a hot bath. Soak in this bath with your entire body—except your head—underwater for as long as possible to reap the full benefits of this detox recipe.

SWAP: This remedy can be made with 20 drops of either lavender or tea tree essential oil if you're out of one or the other.

Low Energy Aid Inhalation Blend

Scent: MINTY AND CITRUSY *Makes:* 1 INHALER
Direct Inhalation: SAFE FOR AGES 10+

If you're feeling sluggish and low on energy, this blend can help you recharge. Invigorating and stimulating peppermint essential oil dances with uplifting and energizing lemongrass essential oil to create an effectively rousing remedy.

2 drops lemongrass essential oil

1 drop peppermint essential oil

Aromatherapy inhaler

2 pipettes

1. Drop the essential oils into the inhaler using the pipettes.

2. Close the cap tightly on the inhaler and take three to five deep breaths of this blend when you need an energy boost.

3. Take a 30-minute break from inhalation.

4. Repeat as needed throughout the day.

SWAP: If you are out of peppermint essential oil, you can substitute spearmint or eucalyptus oil.

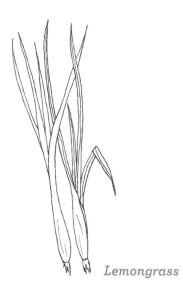

Lemongrass

A Treat for Sore Feet Massage Blend

Scent: MINTY AND HERBACEOUS *Makes:* 1 OUNCE
Topical Application: SAFE FOR AGES 10+

When you have been standing or walking for long periods of time, your feet will usually let you know. On days when you get home and your feet are tender and sore, try this foot massage blend for soothing relief.

Small funnel

1-ounce tinted glass
   bottle with lid

1 ounce carrier oil of
   your choice

6 drops peppermint
   essential oil

6 drops Roman
   chamomile
   essential oil

2 pipettes

1. Place the funnel on the open bottle and pour in the carrier oil. Remove the funnel.

2. Add the essential oils using the pipettes.

3. Close the cap tightly and shake the bottle gently to blend the oils.

4. Apply a quarter-size drop on each foot, massaging thoroughly into the entire foot, including the bottom, heel, toes, top, ankle, and calf, until the oil is absorbed into the skin.

SWAP: Do not use peppermint essential oil on children younger than six. Make sure to keep all remedies out of the reach of young children.

Agony of the Feet Arthritis and Gout Foot Soak

Scent: HERBACEOUS AND FRESH *Makes:* 1 LITER (ENOUGH FOR ONE TREATMENT)
Topical Application: SAFE FOR AGES 10+

When your feet are showing signs of arthritis or gout, this powerful foot soak treatment can help relieve pain, soreness, irritation, and spasms. The oils in this recipe stimulate circulation and lessen inflammation.

Large container to soak feet (needs to hold at least 1 liter of water)

1 liter warm water

Small container to mix oils and castile soap

10 drops Roman chamomile essential oil

8 drops ginger essential oil

8 drops rosemary essential oil

8 drops frankincense essential oil

1 tablespoon unscented castile soap

1. Set the large container in the bathtub to prevent spillage or messes on the floor. Fill the container with 1 liter of warm water.

2. In the small container, mix the essential oils with the unscented castile soap, then pour into the water, making sure to blend everything well.

3. Sit on the edge of the tub with your feet in the container.

4. Agitate the water with your feet to blend the oils during the treatment.

5. Enjoy until the water cools.

TIP: Add ½ cup Epsom salts to this recipe for additional healing.

Well Heeled Moisturizing Massage Blend

Scent: FLORAL AND HERBACEOUS *Makes:* 1 OUNCE
Topical Application: SAFE FOR AGES 6+

The heels often become dry and cracked, especially in the winter months. This recipe can help nourish and soothe heels that need moisture. Geranium and lavender essential oils are famous for relieving dry, irritated skin.

Small funnel

1-ounce tinted glass bottle with lid

¾ ounce avocado oil

6 drops geranium essential oil

6 drops lavender essential oil

2 pipettes

1 pair breathable socks

1. Place the funnel on the bottle and pour in the avocado oil. Remove the funnel.

2. Add the essential oils using the pipettes.

3. Close the cap tightly and shake the bottle gently to blend the oils.

4. Apply a liberal amount of this oil blend to the heels before bed and then put on a pair of socks to contain the oils while sleeping.

5. Repeat nightly for best results.

SWAP: Frankincense essential oil makes an excellent substitute for geranium in this blend.

Nail Nourishment Antifungal Blend

Scent: MEDICINAL AND CITRUSY *Makes:* 1 OUNCE
Topical Application: SAFE FOR AGES 6+

This treatment is perfect for those suffering from fungal issues of the nails, whether on the hands or the feet. Tea tree and lemon essential oils are antifungal and cleansing, so they kill the fungus causing problems and heal any lingering damage. This blend also works well for treating ringworm. Remember, lemon essential oil is phototoxic, so don't expose your hands and feet to sunlight after applying this remedy.

Small funnel
1-ounce tinted glass
   bottle with lid
1 ounce melted
   coconut oil
10 drops tea tree
   essential oil
8 drops lemon
   essential oil
2 pipettes
1 pair gloves or socks
   (depending on what
   you are treating)
2 pipettes

1. Place the funnel on the bottle and pour in the melted coconut oil. Remove the funnel.

2. Add the essential oils using the pipettes.

3. Close the cap tightly and shake the bottle gently to blend the oils.

4. Apply a quarter-size drop to the hands or feet before bed to combat fungus. After applying the oil blend to your feet, put on a pair of socks to contain the oils. If applying to the hands at bedtime, put on gloves to prevent getting the oils on bedsheets, pillows, etc.

5. Repeat nightly for best results.

SWAP: Clove essential oil can replace either oil in this recipe, but make sure to reduce the amount to four or five drops.

Curb Your Cravings Diffusion Blend

Scent: MINTY AND FRUITY *Makes:* ENOUGH FOR MULTIPLE 20-MINUTE DIFFUSIONS
Inhalation via Atmospheric Diffusion: SAFE FOR AGES 6+

If you are struggling with cravings for unhealthy foods and snacks, this blend can help curb the appetite and stimulate the senses to redirect your impulses. The invigorating combination of grapefruit and peppermint essential oils has been shown to reduce cravings and control an overactive appetite.

Ultrasonic diffuser

3 ounces water

5 drops peppermint essential oil

5 drops grapefruit essential oil

1. Fill an ultrasonic diffuser with the water.

2. Add the essential oils and turn on the diffuser.

3. Run the diffuser for 15 to 20 minutes to enjoy the therapeutic benefits. Turn off the diffuser.

4. Repeat after one hour, if needed.

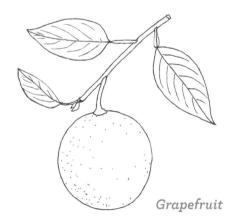

Grapefruit

In the Zone Diffusion Blend

Scent: MINTY *Makes:* ENOUGH FOR MULTIPLE 20-MINUTE DIFFUSIONS
Inhalation via Atmospheric Diffusion: SAFE FOR AGES 10+

When you need to get in the zone before a strenuous workout, this blend can give you the boost of energy you need to reach your full potential. The combination of peppermint and eucalyptus essential oils stimulates the senses and the body in preparation for any training you decide to take on.

Ultrasonic diffuser

3 ounces water

5 drops peppermint essential oil

5 drops eucalyptus essential oil

1. Fill an ultrasonic diffuser with the water.

2. Add the essential oils and turn on the diffuser.

3. Run the diffuser for 10 minutes before starting your workout. (If possible, set the timer to go off 10 minutes into the workout.) Turn off the diffuser.

SWAP: If you are out of either peppermint or eucalyptus essential oil, try substituting spearmint or tea tree oil.

Cool Down Inhalation Blend

Scent: FLORAL AND EARTHY *Makes:* 1 INHALER
Direct Inhalation: SAFE FOR AGES 6+

When your workout has ended and it's time to calm the body, this blend of lavender, bergamot, and patchouli essential oils can help bring your mind and body back to a normal pace. These oils work together to promote a healthy heart rate and a positive outlook.

1 drop lavender essential oil

1 drop bergamot essential oil

1 drop patchouli essential oil

Aromatherapy inhaler

3 pipettes

1. Drop the essential oils into the inhaler using the pipettes.
2. Close the cap tightly on the inhaler and take three to five deep breaths of this blend following your workout.
3. Take a 15-minute break from inhalation.
4. Repeat as needed to help the body wind down and the pulse return to normal.

SWAP: Frankincense, cedarwood, or vetiver essential oils make great substitutes for patchouli in this blend.

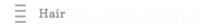

Delousing Mask Treatment

Scent: MEDICINAL *Makes:* 1 CUP
Topical Application: SAFE FOR AGES 5+

As if finding out you or your child has lice isn't stressful enough, most people are led to believe the only effective treatment uses toxic pesticides and chemicals on the head. Most commercial lice products contain ingredients that damage the hair and scalp, but there are other options. Tea tree essential oil is a strong louse repellent and is also very effective in lice prevention. Combining it with coconut oil will smother the lice and prevent them from returning.

1 cup melted coconut oil
Medium mixing bowl
25 drops tea tree
     essential oil (10 drops
     if using on a child)
Spoon
Plastic wrap or shower
     cap (optional)

1. Pour the melted coconut oil into the mixing bowl.

2. Add the tea tree essential oil to the coconut oil and blend thoroughly.

3. Apply a generous amount of the treatment to the scalp and hair as soon as you discover lice. Make sure the scalp and hair are completely coated. If desired, wrap your hair and scalp in plastic wrap or use a shower cap to contain the oil and prevent any lice from escaping the treatment. Keep this treatment on your head for one to two hours. Wash it off in the shower with shampoo as usual. Repeat, if necessary, until no lice or eggs are visible. You may have to use a lice comb or pick the eggs out of the hair.

4. You can also use this treatment for prevention. Leave the treatment on the scalp for 15 minutes, then wash it off in the shower with shampoo as usual.

STORAGE TIP: If you have any of this treatment left over, you can store it in a cool, dark place for as long as the coconut oil is good.

Heal Your Scalp Dandruff Treatment

Scent: HERBACEOUS *Makes:* 1 TABLESPOON
Topical Application: SAFE FOR AGES 10+

When dandruff on the scalp becomes a noticeable problem, essential oils like rosemary and tea tree can help soothe and nourish the scalp while halting the issues that cause dandruff. Rosemary essential oil can help provide gentle circulation to the scalp, while tea tree oil can get rid of any fungal infection that may be contributing to the condition. Grapeseed oil makes a great carrier oil for this treatment because it is light and won't clog pores.

Small funnel

1-ounce tinted glass bottle with lid

1 tablespoon grapeseed oil

3 drops rosemary essential oil

3 drops tea tree essential oil

2 pipettes

1. Place the funnel on the open bottle and pour in the carrier oil. Remove the funnel.

2. Add the essential oils using the pipettes.

3. Close the cap tightly and shake the bottle gently to blend the oils.

4. Apply a quarter-size drop to the scalp and massage thoroughly until absorbed into the skin. Leave the treatment on the scalp for 20 minutes before showering.

5. Use once daily to combat dandruff.

STORAGE TIPS: Any leftover treatment can be stored in a cool, dark place out of the reach of children. Make sure to document the expiration on the grapeseed oil, because this is when the blend expires, too.

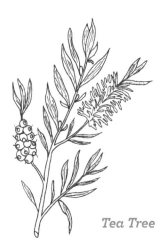

Tea Tree

Migraine Defense Inhalation Blend

Scent: HERBACEOUS AND MINTY *Makes:* 1 INHALER
Direct Inhalation: SAFE FOR AGES 6+

When a headache has you down, this blend can help take the edge off. Peppermint and lavender essential oils are two of the most popular headache remedies because of their ability to ease pain, relax the body, and ease the tension that contributes to some headaches and migraines.

2 drops peppermint essential oil
1 drop lavender essential oil
Aromatherapy inhaler
2 pipettes

1. Drop the essential oils into the inhaler using the pipettes.
2. Close the cap tightly on the inhaler.
3. At the first signs of a headache or migraine, take three to five deep breaths of this blend.
4. Take a 15-minute break from inhalation.
5. Repeat until the migraine or headache has subsided.

TIP: Adding one drop of tea tree essential oil may enhance the therapeutic effects of this blend.

Pacify Menstrual Symptoms Diffusion Blend

Scent: FRUITY AND HERBACEOUS
Makes: ENOUGH FOR MULTIPLE 20-MINUTE DIFFUSIONS
Inhalation via Atmospheric Diffusion: SAFE FOR AGES 8+

Symptoms of premenstrual syndrome include mood swings, cramping, acne, tender breasts, irritability, and fatigue. Many women suffer from these undesirable side effects of pre-period hormones. The essential oils in this blend may help provide calm, clarity, peace, pain relief, balance, and uplift during this time.

Ultrasonic diffuser

3 ounces water

5 drops clary sage essential oil

3 drops cedarwood essential oil

3 drops bergamot essential oil

1. Fill an ultrasonic diffuser with the water.

2. Add the essential oils and turn on the diffuser.

3. Run the diffuser for 20 to 30 minutes in a room where you can be alone to meditate and relax. Turn off the diffuser.

4. Repeat after one hour, if needed.

Hormone Helper Roller Blend

Scent: EARTHY AND HERBACEOUS *Makes:* 10 MILLILITERS
Topical Application: SAFE FOR AGES 12+

When hormones fluctuate and cause issues like mood swings, irregular periods, and acne, this blend can balance and nurture the body. A combination of balancing and calming essential oils like clary sage, lavender, and patchouli is perfect for promoting hormonal stability.

Small funnel

10-milliliter tinted glass
   roller bottle

9 milliliters (about
   2 teaspoons) carrier
   oil of your choice

3 drops lavender
   essential oil

3 drops patchouli
   essential oil

6 drops clary sage
   essential oil

3 pipettes

1. Place the funnel on the open roller bottle and pour in the carrier oil. Remove the funnel.

2. Drop the essential oils into the roller bottle using the pipettes.

3. Firmly place the roller top and cap back on the bottle. Shake the bottle gently to blend the oils.

4. Apply a small amount to the inner thigh (switching sides each application) twice daily for hormonal support.

SWAP: Vetiver or cedarwood essential oil will work well as a substitute for patchouli in this blend.

Cool It Now Spray

Scent: MINTY *Makes:* 1 OUNCE
Topical Application: SAFE FOR AGES 10+

Hot flashes can be an uncomfortable part of menopause for many people. They feel like a sudden flush of heat coming over the body and last several minutes to several hours. Help cool down the body with this invigorating and refreshing spray.

Small funnel

1-ounce tinted glass spray bottle

¼ ounce aloe vera juice

½ ounce distilled water

6 drops clary sage essential oil

10 drops peppermint essential oil

2 pipettes

1. Place the funnel on the bottle and pour in the distilled water and aloe vera juice. Remove the funnel.

2. Add the essential oils using the pipettes.

3. Firmly secure the spray cap on the bottle.

4. Shake vigorously before each use, as the essential oils will separate from the water and float on top. Apply to the arms, legs, chest, and abdomen during a hot flash. Avoid spraying in the eyes or mucous membranes.

5. Repeat as often as needed during hot flashes.

TIP: 1 to 2 drops of bergamot essential oil make a great addition to this blend. Just make sure to stay out of direct sunlight if you add this oil.

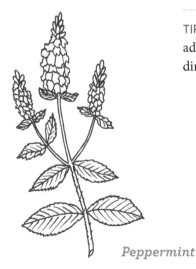
Peppermint

Don't Let It Cramp Your Style Massage Blend

Scent: HERBACEOUS *Makes:* 1 OUNCE
Topical Application: SAFE FOR AGES 10+

Menstrual cramps can be brutal, but essential oils that relieve pain and muscle spasms can take the edge off. Roman chamomile essential oil is antispasmodic and analgesic, making it ideal for cramp relief. Clary sage is known as a "women's herb" because of its ability to help relieve uterine contractions and soothe muscles.

Small funnel

1-ounce tinted glass bottle with lid

1 ounce carrier oil of your choice

10 drops clary sage essential oil

10 drops Roman chamomile essential oil

2 pipettes

1. Place the funnel on the bottle and pour in the carrier oil. Remove the funnel.

2. Add the essential oils using the pipettes.

3. Close the cap tightly and shake the bottle gently to blend the oils.

4. When you are experiencing menstrual cramping, apply a quarter-size drop to the lower abdominal area over the uterus and massage into the skin thoroughly. Use a heating pad afterward to further relieve cramping and soothe the uterus.

TLC for Psoriasis and Eczema Roller Blend

Scent: EARTHY *Makes:* 10 MILLILITERS
Topical Application: SAFE FOR AGES 6+

Eczema and psoriasis can be painful and distracting. Both conditions involve irritated, itchy skin that appears in patches on various areas of the body. When skin needs some serious nourishment and moisture, this blend of frankincense, lavender, and patchouli essential oils can work wonders. The avocado oil in this recipe helps further soothe skin, as well as provide skin with vitamins and minerals to help repair damage.

Small funnel
10-milliliter tinted glass roller bottle
9 milliliters (about 2 teaspoons) avocado oil
3 drops lavender essential oil
4 drops frankincense essential oil
3 drops patchouli essential oil
3 pipettes

1. Place the funnel on the open roller bottle and pour in the avocado oil. Remove the funnel.

2. Drop the essential oils into the roller bottle using the pipettes.

3. Firmly place the roller top and cap back on the bottle. Shake the bottle gently to blend the oils.

4. Apply the contents of the bottle directly to the affected areas, massaging in any excess oils.

5. Repeat up to twice daily for best results.

Inflammation Fighter Roller Blend

Scent: EARTHY *Makes:* 10 MILLILITERS
Topical Application: SAFE FOR AGES 5+

Inflammation of the skin can look like raised, red, irritated patches. It can also show up as swollen, tender areas. Inflammation usually results from a histamine reaction under the skin caused by contact with allergens or irritants. Other causes include autoimmune issues, where the body's immune system attacks itself. Whatever the cause, essential oils like frankincense and lavender can help reduce inflammation, soothe irritated skin, provide antioxidants, and counter histamine reactions.

Small funnel
10-milliliter tinted glass
   roller bottle
9 milliliters (about
   2 teaspoons) carrier
   oil of your choice
5 drops frankincense
   essential oil
5 drops lavender
   essential oil
2 pipettes

1. Place the funnel on the open roller bottle and pour in the carrier oil. Remove the funnel.

2. Drop the essential oils into the roller bottle using the pipettes.

3. Firmly place the roller top and cap back on the bottle. Shake the bottle gently to blend the oils.

4. Apply this blend to areas that are swollen, tender, inflamed, red, or irritated to provide soothing relief. This blend also works great for inflammation caused by insect stings and bites.

TIP: Adding one or two drops of tea tree essential oil can enhance the healing effects of this remedy.

Nix the Itch Roller Blend

Scent: HERBACEOUS *Makes:* 10 MILLILITERS
Topical Application: SAFE FOR AGES 5+

Itching can lead to serious issues such as infection or excoriation of the skin. When you are plagued with itchy skin, this blend can ease your discomfort and help the area heal. Lavender, frankincense, and tea tree essential oils combine to provide relief and promote skin recovery.

Small funnel
10-milliliter tinted glass roller bottle
8 milliliters carrier oil of your choice
10 drops lavender essential oil
10 drops tea tree essential oil
6 drops frankincense essential oil
3 pipettes

1. Place the funnel on the open roller bottle and pour in the carrier oil. Remove the funnel.
2. Drop the essential oils into the roller bottle using the pipettes.
3. Firmly place the roller top and cap back on the bottle. Shake the bottle gently to blend the oils.
4. Apply this to areas that are itching or irritated as often as needed.

SWAP: Clary sage essential oil can substitute for frankincense in this blend.

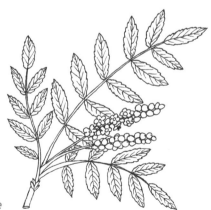

Frankincense

Muscle Miracle Massage Blend

Scent: HERBACEOUS AND CAMPHOROUS *Makes:* 1 OUNCE
Topical Application: SAFE FOR AGES 10+

If sore muscles are affecting your daily routine, it may be time to give them this soothing treatment. Rosemary and peppermint essential oils combine in this blend to aid circulation, relieve pain, and calm tired muscles.

Small funnel

1-ounce tinted glass bottle with lid

¾ ounce carrier oil of your choice

8 drops rosemary essential oil

8 drops peppermint essential oil

2 pipettes

1. Place the funnel on the open bottle and pour in the carrier oil. Remove the funnel.
2. Add the essential oils using the pipettes.
3. Close the cap tightly and shake the bottle gently to blend the oils.
4. Apply a small amount of this blend to the areas where you are experiencing soreness and massage it into the skin until the oils are absorbed.
5. Repeat daily, as needed, for the treatment of sore muscles. Avoid getting this blend in open wounds or mucous membranes.

TIPS: Adding wintergreen essential oil can help sore muscles as well. This is very strong, so use only one to two drops.

Pain in the Neck Roller Blend

Scent: HERBACEOUS AND MINTY *Makes:* 1 TABLESPOON
Topical Application: SAFE FOR AGES 6+

Sometimes stress can cause major tension in the neck and back. When this happens, try using this blend to reduce stress as well as the pain and stiffness that result from carrying it. The combination of peppermint and lavender essential oils helps soothe and relax tense muscles.

Small funnel
15-milliliter tinted glass
   roller bottle
1 teaspoon carrier oil
   of your choice
10 drops lavender
   essential oil
8 drops peppermint
   essential oil
2 pipettes

1. Place the funnel on the open bottle and pour in the carrier oil. Remove the funnel.
2. Drop the essential oils into the roller bottle using the pipettes.
3. Firmly place the roller top and cap back on the bottle. Shake the bottle gently to blend the oils.
4. When you are experiencing tension in the back and neck, apply the roller bottle to the areas that need relief and massage thoroughly until the oil is absorbed.
5. Repeat up to two times daily for relief.

SWAP: You can use Roman chamomile or clary sage essential oil as a substitute for either oil in this blend.

Gas Relief Massage Blend

Scent: FRESH AND MINTY *Makes:* 1 OUNCE
Topical Application: SAFE FOR AGES 6+

When gas and bloating have you feeling less than stellar, try massaging this powerful blend into your stomach for relief. Peppermint and ginger essential oils both have carminative and digestive properties, making them wonderful for helping alleviate painful gas and bloating.

Small funnel
1-ounce tinted glass
   bottle with lid
¾ ounce carrier oil of
   your choice
6 drops peppermint
   essential oil
10 drops ginger
   essential oil
2 pipettes

1. Place the funnel on the open bottle and pour in the carrier oil. Remove the funnel.

2. Add the essential oils using the pipettes.

3. Close the cap tightly and shake the bottle gently to blend the oils.

4. When you experience gas, bloating, and related discomfort in the abdomen, apply a quarter-size drop of this blend to the area on the stomach where you feel discomfort. Massage the area thoroughly until the oils have absorbed into the skin. Lie on your side for at least 20 minutes, as this can also help relieve the discomfort. If you have a heating pad, try applying heat to the area as well.

5. Repeat as needed for relief from gas and bloating.

SWAP: For a more kid-friendly blend, use spearmint essential oil instead of peppermint.

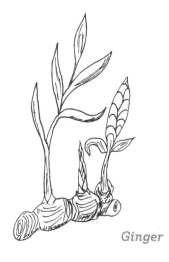
Ginger

Indigestion Rescue Roller Blend

Scent: HERBACEOUS AND FRESH *Makes:* 10 MILLILITERS
Topical Application: SAFE FOR AGES 6+

Indigestion can be painful. It usually occurs when you have eaten a big meal or something that doesn't agree with you. You might have experience very "full" feeling, heartburn, nausea, or pain. Essential oils can help calm the storm and prevent the spasms that cause pain and nausea.

Small funnel

10-milliliter tinted glass
   roller bottle

9 milliliters (about
   2 teaspoons) carrier
   oil of your choice

10 drops Roman
   chamomile
   essential oil

6 drops peppermint
   essential oil

6 drops ginger
   essential oil

3 pipettes

1. Place the funnel on the open roller bottle and pour in the carrier oil. Remove the funnel.

2. Drop the essential oils into the roller bottle using the pipettes.

3. Firmly place the roller top and cap back on the bottle. Shake the bottle gently to blend the oils.

4. When you are experiencing symptoms of indigestion, apply the roller bottle to the stomach where you are experiencing discomfort. Massage the oils into the skin. Sit up to prevent more heartburn or discomfort, and use a heating pad if necessary.

5. Repeat as needed when you have indigestion.

Knock Out Nausea Motion Sickness Inhalation Blend

Scent: FRESH *Makes:* 1 INHALER
Direct Inhalation: SAFE FOR AGES 6+

This inhalation blend is ideal for those who suffer from car sickness, motion sickness, vertigo, and morning sickness. It can help alleviate the symptoms of nausea and settle the stomach. This is a great remedy to add to a travel bag.

1 drop peppermint essential oil

2 drops ginger essential oil

Aromatherapy inhaler

2 pipettes

1. Drop the essential oils into the inhaler using the pipettes.

2. Close the cap tightly on the inhaler and take three to five deep breaths of this blend when you are experiencing nausea. Keep your eyes fixed on an immovable object and focus on your breathing.

3. Take a 10- to 15-minute breaks from inhalation.

4. Repeat as needed throughout the day.

SWAP: Spearmint essential oil is always an effective substitute for peppermint oil.

Keep Clear of Cold Sores Roller Blend

Scent: MEDICINAL AND FRESH *Makes:* 10 MILLILITERS
Topical Application: SAFE FOR AGES 8+

Cold sores are symptoms of a virus that can attack the body, especially when immune defenses are down. Try this powerful blend of ginger, lemon, and tea tree essential oils to combat the effects. Lemon essential oil is phototoxic, so don't use this remedy before sun exposure.

Small funnel
10-milliliter tinted glass
  roller bottle
9 milliliters (about
  2 teaspoons) carrier
  oil of your choice
6 drops tea tree
  essential oil
6 drops lemon
  essential oil
4 drops ginger
  essential oil
3 pipettes

1. Place the funnel on the open roller bottle and pour in the carrier oil. Remove the funnel.

2. Drop the essential oils into the roller bottle using the pipettes.

3. Firmly place the roller top and cap back on the bottle. Shake the bottle gently to blend the oils.

4. Apply a small amount directly to an emerging cold sore to provide relief and healing. The sooner you can start applying this, the more effective it will be. Apply up to four times daily at the first sign of a cold sore. Discontinue use if you notice skin irritation or a skin reaction.

5. Use caution when using this remedy, as the lemon essential oil can cause a reaction if applied before prolonged sun exposure.

TIP: Melissa (lemon balm) is another highly effective essential oil for cold sores. This oil tends to be pricier, but just six drops can be a beneficial addition to this blend.

SAFETY TIP: Lemon essential oil is phototoxic, so don't use this remedy before sun exposure.

Flu Fighters Diffusion Blend

Scent: SPICY *Makes:* ENOUGH FOR MULTIPLE 20-MINUTE DIFFUSIONS
Inhalation via Atmospheric Diffusion: SAFE FOR AGES 10+

When the days get shorter and there is less sunlight to provide critical vitamin D, the immune system can become weaker. To combat viruses that emerge during cold and flu season, try diffusing this blend of clove and cinnamon essential oils, which kill airborne influenza pathogens. This blend is great for cleansing the air when members of your household are ill with a virus.

Ultrasonic diffuser

3 ounces water

5 drops clove
  essential oil

5 drops cinnamon
  essential oil

1. Fill an ultrasonic diffuser with the water.

2. Add the essential oils and turn on the diffuser.

3. Run the diffuser for 20 minutes. Turn off the diffuser. You can then either take it to another room and run it for and additional 20 minutes or keep it in your main living area.

4. Repeat daily when viruses are present in the household.

SWAP: Other great essential oils to use during cold and flu season include lemon balm, rosemary, eucalyptus, tea tree, oregano, thyme, and peppermint. Try any of these as a substitute for the oils in this blend.

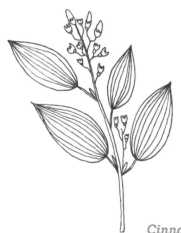

Cinnamon

Kid-Safe Clear the Air Blend

Scent: HERBACEOUS AND FRUITY
Makes: ENOUGH FOR MULTIPLE 20-MINUTE DIFFUSIONS
Inhalation via Atmospheric Diffusion: SAFE FOR AGES 5+

Some antiviral blends are unsafe for children, especially those containing the constituent 1,8 cineole. You can avoid these oils and still combat viruses with this powerful blend of tea tree and lemon essential oils.

Ultrasonic diffuser
3 ounces water
5 drops tea tree
   essential oil
4 drops lemon
   essential oil

1. Fill an ultrasonic diffuser with the water.
2. Add the essential oils.
3. Turn on this diffuser in your child's room (or wherever they tend to hang out most when they are sick).
4. Run the diffuser for 15 to 20 minutes. Turn off the diffuser.
5. Repeat after 30 minutes, if needed.

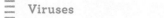 Viruses

Immune Booster Diffusion Blend

Scent: SPICY AND HERBACEOUS
Makes: ENOUGH FOR MULTIPLE 20-MINUTE DIFFUSIONS
Inhalation via Atmospheric Diffusion: SAFE FOR AGES 10+

Some essential oils can help stimulate the immune system, making it easier for your body to fight a virus. Diffuse this blend if you feel a cold or virus coming on, or if you just want a boost.

Ultrasonic diffuser
3 ounces water
3 drops rosemary
essential oil
2 drops clove
essential oil
2 drops tea tree
essential oil
4 drops thyme
essential oil

1. Fill an ultrasonic diffuser with the water.
2. Add the essential oils and turn on the diffuser.
3. Run the diffuser for 20 minutes. Turn off the diffuser.
4. Repeat after 30 minutes to one hour, if needed.

TIP: Although not an essential oil, elderberry is a wonderful immunomodulatory plant and can help tremendously when it comes to combating viruses. Consider adding this to your seasonal health arsenal.

Stay Cool Fever Treatment Compress

Scent: MINTY AND MEDICINAL *Makes:* 1 CUP
Topical Application: SAFE FOR AGES 6+

Fevers are usually a sign of a normally functioning immune system trying to combat a pathogen by killing it with heat. However, in some people, fevers can get very high, and they need treatment to avoid the risk of febrile seizures and related complications. If you are looking for a natural fever reducer, peppermint and tea tree essential oils can help lower the body temperature.

1 cup distilled water

1 tablespoon carrier oil of your choice

16-ounce glass canning jar with lid

10 drops peppermint essential oil

10 drops tea tree essential oil

2 pipettes

1 to 4 small cloths for soaking

1. Pour the water into the jar.

2. Add the essential oils to the carrier oil using the pipettes. Then, add all the oils to the jar.

3. Close the lid and shake well to blend the oil and water. Remove the lid carefully.

4. Add one cloth to the liquid, completely saturating it. Close the lid and shake the contents of the container again. Remove the cloth from the container and wring it out. Continue soaking cloths as needed.

5. Place the cloths on the back of the neck, arms, chest, legs, or forehead (avoid getting the treatment in the eyes!).

6. Leave the cloths on the body until the fever begins to subside. Keep the person with the fever in cool clothing to prevent the body temperature from rising again.

SAFETY TIP: For children under the age of six, use only five drops of tea tree essential oil and omit the peppermint oil.

Unlucky Break Massage Blend

Scent: EARTHY AND HERBACEOUS *Makes:* 1 OUNCE
Topical Application: SAFE FOR AGES 6+

Plants have been used throughout history to heal wounds. Since essential oils are the concentrated product of plants, it is no wonder they are so effective at healing. Roman chamomile and frankincense pair well in this massage blend to nurture fractures and sprains. Both oils are anti-inflammatory and can help reduce trauma.

Small funnel
1-ounce tinted glass bottle with lid
1 ounce olive oil
10 drops frankincense essential oil
10 drops Roman chamomile essential oil
2 pipettes

1. Place the funnel on the open bottle and pour in the olive oil. Remove the funnel.
2. Add the essential oils using the pipettes.
3. Close the cap tightly and shake the bottle gently to blend the oils.
4. When you have experienced trauma like a sprain or fracture, apply a quarter-size drop of this blend to the area and gently massage it into the skin to promote healing.

SAFETY TIP: When using this blend, stay away from open wounds and avoid getting any in or near mucous membranes.

Scar Care Oil

Scent: EARTHY AND FLORAL *Makes:* 10 MILLILITERS
Topical Application: SAFE FOR AGES 6+

If you have a scar that is bothering you, you may find that this blend helps reduce its appearance as well as the inflammation and discoloration. The blend contains three powerful essential oils known for their ability to heal the skin.

Small funnel

10-milliliter tinted glass roller bottle

9 milliliters (about 2 teaspoons) jojoba oil

4 drops geranium essential oil

4 drops patchouli essential oil

8 drops frankincense essential oil

3 pipettes

1. Place the funnel on the open roller bottle and pour in the jojoba oil. Remove the funnel.

2. Drop the essential oils into the roller bottle using the pipettes.

3. Firmly place the roller top and cap back on the bottle. Shake the bottle gently to blend the oils.

4. Apply this blend directly to scars each morning and evening.

SWAP: Lavender essential oil can substitute for geranium oil in this blend.

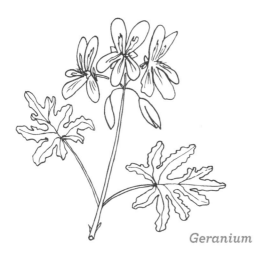

Geranium

Boo-Boo Spray

Scent: MEDICINAL *Makes:* 1 OUNCE
Topical Application: SAFE FOR AGES 5+

The oils in this blend work to cleanse minor wounds, prevent infection, and promote healing. Tea tree essential oil kills bacteria, while lavender essential oil can help relieve skin trauma and soothe. Frankincense oil can nurture the skin and help reduce scarring.

Small funnel
1-ounce tinted glass
  spray bottle
¼ ounce aloe vera juice
½ ounce distilled water
10 drops tea tree
  essential oil
10 drops lavender
  essential oil
5 drops frankincense
  essential oil
3 pipettes

1. Place the funnel on the open bottle and pour in the distilled water and aloe vera juice. Remove the funnel.

2. Add the essential oils using the pipettes.

3. Firmly attach the spray cap to the bottle.

4. Shake vigorously before use. Apply directly to minor cuts and scrapes after washing with soap and water. Allow the area to dry thoroughly before bandaging.

SAFETY TIP: Although this blend is very effective for cleansing minor wounds, avoid using on more serious wounds, as this may cause more irritation to the area. Seek immediate medical attention for anything that will not stop bleeding.

Contusion Conclusion Roller Blend

Scent: FLORAL *Makes:* 10 MILLILITERS
Topical Application: SAFE FOR AGES 6+

Contusions can look and feel bothersome. They are often the result of trauma to the skin. When the skin is injured, small blood vessels can break, causing blood to get trapped in areas under the skin. The area may become sore, tender to the touch, inflamed, irritated, and discolored. Essential oils can promote healing in these areas while reducing inflammation.

Small funnel

10-milliliter tinted glass roller bottle

9 milliliters (about 2 tablespoons) carrier oil of your choice

6 drops geranium essential oil

8 drops lavender essential oil

6 drops frankincense essential oil

3 pipettes

1. Place the funnel on the open roller bottle and pour in the carrier oil. Remove the funnel.

2. Drop the essential oils into the roller bottle using the pipettes.

3. Firmly place the roller top and cap back on the bottle. Shake the bottle gently to blend the oils.

4. Gently apply this blend directly to contusions up to twice daily to promote healing.

SWAP: Roman chamomile essential oil can be used in place of lavender oil in this remedy.

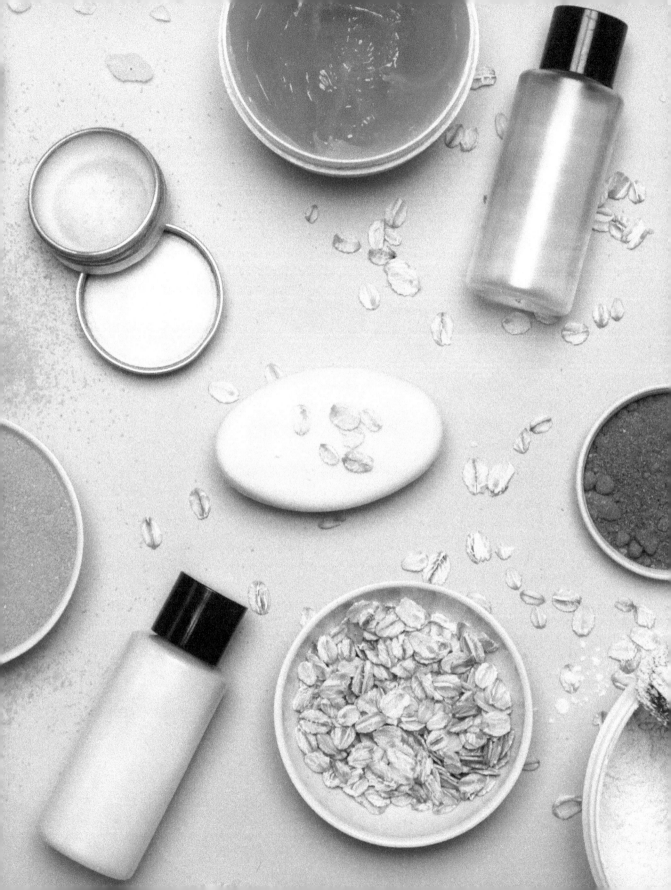

8

BEAUTY AND WELLNESS

The therapeutic powers of essential oils make them a superior alternative to the commercial beauty and wellness products we use each day. Many beauty products contain concerning amounts of toxic substances that have been linked to cancers, hormone issues, and more. Replacing these toxic products with more natural alternatives may have a significant effect on health. What's more, it is surprisingly simple to use essential oils to create your own beauty products.

Bye-Bye Blackheads Acne Treatment Blend

Scent: MEDICINAL AND CITRUSY *Makes:* 1 TABLESPOON
Topical Application: SAFE FOR AGES 8+

Say goodbye to acne and blackheads with this helpful and powerful recipe. Anti-microbial tea tree and bergamot essential oils combine to nourish skin and fight bacteria that contribute to skin eruptions. The light, non-pore-clogging grapeseed carrier oil makes this recipe even more effective.

Small funnel

15-milliliter tinted glass roller bottle

1 tablespoon grapeseed oil

10 drops tea tree essential oil

8 drops bergamot essential oil

2 pipettes

1. Place the funnel on the open roller bottle and pour in the grapeseed oil. Remove the funnel.

2. Drop the essential oils into the roller bottle using the pipettes.

3. Firmly place the roller top and cap back on the bottle. Shake the bottle gently to blend the oils.

4. Apply a small amount directly to the affected areas at bedtime. This can be repeated nightly until the skin clears.

TIP: Adding lavender essential oil to this remedy can help if you have acne accompanied by redness and irritation. Add eight drops for this purpose.

Clean Your Face Makeup Remover

Scent: HERBACEOUS AND FRUITY *Makes:* 1 OUNCE
Topical Application: SAFE FOR AGES 8+

Oil-based commercial makeup removers often contain cheap mineral oil, while others have abrasive and drying ingredients that are not good for the skin. You can create your own simple and effective makeup remover using essential oils like lavender and bergamot. This cleansing recipe removes makeup while nourishing your skin.

Small funnel

1-ounce tinted glass
  bottle with lid

⅓ ounce castor oil

⅔ ounce grapeseed oil

8 drops bergamot
  essential oil

10 drops lavender
  essential oil

2 pipettes

1. Place the funnel on the bottle and pour in the castor and grapeseed oils. Remove the funnel.

2. Add the essential oils using the pipettes.

3. Close the cap tightly and shake the bottle gently to blend the oils.

4. Apply a quarter-size drop to the face and spread evenly, massaging into the skin. Leave on for five minutes before rinsing off with warm water.

5. Repeat as necessary.

SWAP: If you have severely oily skin, skip the castor oil and replace it with more grapeseed oil or sweet.

About Face Oily or Combination Skin Treatment Spray

Scent: MEDICINAL AND HERBACEOUS *Makes:* 1 OUNCE
Topical Application: SAFE FOR AGES 6+

This soothing treatment can help calm red, irritated skin and fight the inflammation that comes with painful acne. The spray bottle also makes it easy to apply. Tea tree and lavender essential oils are known for their skin-soothing and antimicrobial properties, making them ideal for treating oily skin and acne. This recipe is also great for combination skin in need of balance.

Small funnel

1-ounce tinted glass spray bottle

¾ ounce witch hazel extract

10 drops lavender essential oil

10 drops tea tree essential oil

2 pipettes

1. Place the funnel on the bottle and pour in the witch hazel extract. Remove the funnel.

2. Add the essential oils using the pipettes.

3. Firmly secure the spray cap on the bottle.

4. Shake vigorously before use. Carefully apply the spray to the face, avoiding contact with the eyes.

5. Repeat up to three times daily to help control oil and acne.

SWAP: For enhanced bacteria-killing properties, substitute the witch hazel extract for colloidal silver. You can even use half witch hazel and half colloidal silver to benefit from each.

In the Clear Acne Control Mask

Scent: LIGHT CITRUS SCENT *Makes:* 1 TABLESPOON
Topical Application: SAFE FOR AGES 8+

One of the most surprising antimicrobial substances is raw honey. Raw honey collected from beehives will not go bad; in fact, it is one of the most shelf-stable products you can find. Raw honey is amazingly beneficial for the skin and can help soothe, kill bacteria, and promote a healthy glow. Adding bergamot essential oil creates an amazing ultra-nourishing skin treatment for oily and acne-prone skin.

1 tablespoon raw honey
4 drops bergamot
  essential oil
Small mixing bowl
Spoon

1. Combine the honey and bergamot essential oil in the mixing bowl.
2. Spread on the face evenly and liberally. Lie down to prevent drips or spills. Leave the mask on the skin for 20 minutes.
3. Gently rinse off the mask with warm water.
4. Repeat daily to treat and prevent acne.

TIP: Heating honey destroys the therapeutic properties.

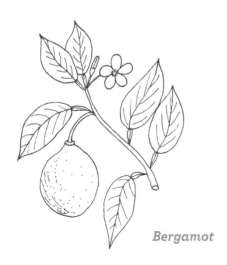

Bergamot

Wrinkle Reducer Anti-Aging Serum

Scent: EARTHY *Makes:* 1 OUNCE
Topical Application: SAFE FOR AGES 10+

This serum is perfect for both wrinkle prevention and treatment. A combination of frankincense and patchouli essential oils helps condition the skin and provide it with antioxidants. These oils can soften and smooth fine lines and support youthful skin. The rosehip carrier oil further enhances this serum's healing properties.

Small funnel
1-ounce tinted glass dropper bottle
1 ounce rosehip oil
10 drops frankincense essential oil
10 drops patchouli essential oil
2 pipettes

1. Place the funnel on the open bottle and pour in the rosehip oil. Remove the funnel.
2. Add the essential oils using the pipettes.
3. Firmly secure the dropper cap on the bottle and shake well to blend the oils.
4. Apply one dropperful to the face every night at bedtime to promote healthy skin.

SWAP: Jojoba oil is a great substitute for rosehip oil in this blend.

Anti-Aging

Out, Out Age Spot Treatment

Scent: FRUITY AND EARTHY *Makes:* 10 MILLILITERS
Topical Application: SAFE FOR AGES 10+

Age spots are discolorations that appear on the skin. When they begin to appear on the face, you can combat them with this brightening and nourishing recipe. A combination of cleansing and soothing oils like lavender, lemon, and frankincense work together to reduce the appearance of age spots and promote an even complexion.

Small funnel
10-milliliter tinted glass
    roller bottle
9 milliliters (or about
    2 teaspoons)
    jojoba oil
4 drops lemon
    essential oil
6 drops frankincense
    essential oil
6 drops lavender
    essential oil
3 pipettes

1. Place the funnel on the open roller bottle and pour in the jojoba oil. Remove the funnel.
2. Drop the essential oils into the roller bottle using the pipettes.
3. Firmly place the roller top and cap back on the bottle. Shake the bottle gently to blend the oils.
4. Apply this directly to age spots up to two times daily to help reduce their appearance. Use this recipe on a clean face for best results.

SWAP: Geranium essential oil can be used in place of lavender oil in this blend.

SAFETY TIP: Lemon essential oil is phototoxic, so don't use this treatment before sun exposure.

Youthful Glow Mask Treatment

Scent: EARTHY *Makes:* 1 TABLESPOON
Topical Application: SAFE FOR AGES 8+

This skin-nourishing remedy can promote healthy skin, reduce the signs of aging, and provide the skin with deep hydration. Frankincense essential oil and olive oil help hydrate and smooth the skin, while bentonite clay helps pull out any impurities. Oat flour reduces inflammation.

1 teaspoon olive oil

Small mixing bowl

4 drops frankincense
    essential oil

Spoon

1 teaspoon
    bentonite clay

½ teaspoon oat flour
    or instant oatmeal

½ teaspoon water
    (add less or more
    to achieve paste
    consistency)

1. Pour the olive oil into the mixing bowl.

2. Add the frankincense essential oil and mix well.

3. Add the bentonite clay and oat flour and blend thoroughly.

4. Gradually add the water until a paste-like consistency is reached (add a small amount of additional water, if needed).

5. Spread this mixture evenly on the face and leave it on for 20 minutes.

6. Gently rinse off the mask with warm water.

7. Repeat daily for best results.

Full Steam Ahead Facial Treatment

Scent: EARTHY *Makes:* 2 CUPS
Atmospheric Diffusion: SAFE FOR AGES 18+

Frankincense is one of the most popular anti-aging essential oils on the market—and for good reason. This powerful essential oil has been shown to help protect skin cells, tighten the skin, and moisturize. When applied in a steam treatment, frankincense essential oil can work more efficiently because the steam helps open the pores, allowing the airborne oils to penetrate more deeply into the skin.

2 cups water
Small saucepan
Large bowl
10 drops frankincense
    essential oil
1 towel

1. Pour the water into the saucepan and bring it to a boil on the stove.

2. Remove the water from the heat and carefully pour it into the large bowl.

3. Add the frankincense essential oil.

4. Place your face over the steaming bowl (at a safe distance to avoid steam burning).

5. Place a towel over your head to trap the steam.

6. Enjoy this treatment for 10 to 20 minutes.

7. Repeat up to three times a week for best results.

SAFETY TIP: Always use caution when working with hot and steaming water. When placing your face over the bowl, keep it at least 12 inches to avoid a steam burn.

Bright Eyes Dark Circle Treatment

Scent: EARTHY AND FRUITY *Makes:* 10 MILLILITERS
Topical Application: SAFE FOR AGES 10+

Dark circles don't always come from fatigue. They can be genetic, or the result of too much straining, the aging process, or even allergies. Essential oils can help lessen the appearance of these dark circles. In addition to this remedy, try to figure out the underlying cause to help treat the root of the issue.

Small funnel

10-milliliter tinted glass
   roller bottle

9 milliliters (about
   2 teaspoons)
   jojoba oil

6 drops frankincense
   essential oil

4 drops bergamot
   essential oil

2 pipettes

1. Place the funnel on the open roller bottle and pour in the jojoba oil. Remove the funnel.

2. Drop the essential oils into the roller bottle using the pipettes.

3. Firmly place the roller top and cap back on the bottle. Shake the bottle gently to blend the oils.

4. Apply to the under-eye region up to twice daily for best results. Apply only a small amount under the eyes.

SAFETY TIPS: Bergamot essential oil is phototoxic, so don't apply this treatment before sun exposure. Avoid getting this blend in the eyes, as it can cause irritation.

Invigorating Natural Deodorant Body Spray

Scent: MINTY AND CITRUSY *Makes:* 2 OUNCES
Topical Application: SAFE FOR AGES 8+

Synthetic fragrances found in most commercial deodorants simply mask odors. Essential oils can actually help combat the bacteria that create the smell in the first place. Using essential oils in a natural deodorant is a great way to smell amazing while nourishing your skin. The peppermint essential oil in this recipe also cools the underarms, minimizing the chance of developing unwelcome odors.

Small funnel

2-ounce tinted glass
   spray bottle

¾ ounce witch
   hazel extract

½ ounce colloidal silver

½ ounce lavender
   hydrosol or
   distilled water

10 drops peppermint
   essential oil

12 drops lemongrass
   essential oil

2 pipettes

1. Place the funnel on the open bottle and pour in the witch hazel extract, colloidal silver, and lavender hydrosol. Remove the funnel.

2. Add the essential oils using the pipettes.

3. Firmly secure the spray cap on the bottle.

4. Shake vigorously before use. Apply to the armpits.

5. Apply as needed throughout the day to help with odor control.

SWAP: Lavender essential oil can be used in place of peppermint to help provide odor relief, especially if you have sensitive skin.

Skin-Soothing Deodorant

Scent: FLORAL *Makes:* 1 CUP
Topical Application: SAFE FOR AGES 8+

When you make your own deodorant with essential oils, you can create something that actually nurtures the skin in addition to preventing body odor. This recipe uses naturally antimicrobial lavender essential oil, as well as other soothing ingredients, to prevent odor while promoting healthy skin.

Medium mixing bowl
Spoon
⅔ cup melted coconut oil
10 drops lavender essential oil
⅓ cup shea butter
2 tablespoons arrowroot flour
1 tablespoon cornstarch
1 cup container with lid

1. In the mixing bowl, combine the melted coconut oil and lavender essential oil. Mix until blended.

2. Melt the shea butter and add it to the oils.

3. Stir in the arrowroot flour.

4. Stir in the cornstarch until well blended.

5. Transfer the mixture to a container with a lid for storage.

6. Massage a small amount into the armpits daily as needed for odor control.

Armpit Detox Mask

Scent: FLORAL *Makes:* 2 TABLESPOONS
Topical Application: SAFE FOR AGES 10+

Because the armpits are near a large lymphatic gland, impurities that cause body odor can build up. If you notice your body odor worsening, this armpit detox mask may be just what you need. It uses lavender essential oil for its antimicrobial and skin-nurturing abilities.

2 tablespoons bentonite clay
Small mixing bowl
Water (enough to create a paste-like consistency)
Spoon
6 drops lavender essential oil

1. Put the bentonite clay into the mixing bowl.
2. Gradually add small amounts of water, around ½ teaspoon at a time, until the clay becomes paste-like.
3. Add the lavender essential oil and mix well.
4. Apply the mixture evenly to each clean armpit. Leave it on for 20 to 30 minutes before rinsing off with warm water.
5. Repeat once a week for best results.
6. To avoid recontamination of the armpits, try using the deodorant recipes in this book as opposed to commercial products.

SWAP: Tea tree essential oil can substitute for lavender essential oil in this blend.

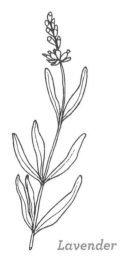

Lavender

Healthy Hair After-Shower Hair Nourishment Spray

Scent: FLORAL AND EARTHY *Makes:* 1 OUNCE
Topical Application: SAFE FOR AGES 6+

To treat or prevent hair issues like split ends, damage, or brittleness, try this rejuvenating recipe. This hair spray contains two of the best essential oils for hair health: patchouli and lavender. Together, they can help nourish hair and heal damage. Apple cider vinegar is also excellent for hair health and makes a great addition to this recipe.

Small funnel

1-ounce tinted glass spray bottle

5 teaspoons distilled water

1 teaspoon raw unfiltered apple cider vinegar

8 drops lavender essential oil

8 drops patchouli essential oil

2 pipettes

1. Place the funnel on the open bottle and pour in the water and apple cider vinegar. Remove the funnel.

2. Add the essential oils using the pipettes.

3. Firmly secure the spray cap on the bottle.

4. Shake vigorously before use. Spritz onto towel-dried hair once or twice after showering.

5. Repeat daily, or as often as you shower, for best results.

TIP: For additional nourishment, you can infuse herbs like stinging nettle or calendula into the apple cider vinegar before using it in the remedy. To do this, simply fill a jar with herbs and completely cover with apple cider vinegar. Leave it in a cool, dark place for one month, shaking daily to help infuse. Strain it before use.

Hair Help Damage Repair Mask

Scent: FLORAL *Makes:* 1 CUP
Topical Application: SAFE FOR AGES 8+

A combination of hair-nourishing carrier oils and essential oils makes this mask wonderful for hair restoration and repair. Coconut oil replenishes and hydrates, while jojoba oil helps lock in moisture and restore hair in need of help. Lavender and geranium essential oils repair current damage while preventing future harm.

½ cup melted coconut oil

8-ounce container with lid

½ jojoba oil

10 drops lavender essential oil

10 drops geranium essential oil

1. Pour the melted coconut oil into the container.
2. Add the jojoba oil.
3. Add the essential oils.
4. Secure the lid on the container and shake gently to blend the oils.
5. Apply liberally to clean, dry hair. Massage into the hair. Go easy on the scalp and top of the head. Leave the hair mask on for 20 minutes.
6. To rinse off, shower as usual. Repeat shampooing, if needed, to get all the oil out of the hair.

STORAGE TIP: This recipe provides enough hair mask treatment to last several months. Store it in a cool, dark place and label accordingly. The coconut oil will likely be the first to expire in this recipe.

Tress Finesse Hair Growth Mask

Scent: HERBACEOUS *Makes:* 2 OUNCES
Topical Application: SAFE FOR AGES 10+

Have you ever regretted a haircut? Maybe your hair doesn't grow as fast as it once did. Whatever the case, this wonderful recipe can help stimulate scalp circulation and promote hair growth.

Small funnel

2-ounce tinted
  glass bottle

1 tablespoon castor oil

1 tablespoon jojoba oil

6 drops rosemary
  essential oil

1 pipette

1. Place the funnel on the open bottle and pour in the castor oil and jojoba oil. Remove the funnel.

2. Add the rosemary essential oil using the pipette.

3. Firmly place the roller top and cap back on the bottle. Shake the bottle gently to blend the oils.

4. Apply a small amount to the scalp and massage into the skin for five minutes. Leave the treatment on the scalp for another 10 minutes before rinsing off.

5. Repeat daily for best results.

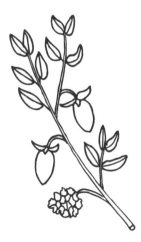

Jojoba oil

Natural Nourishment Conditioner

Scent: EARTHY *Makes:* 1 CUP
Topical Application: SAFE FOR AGES 8+

You can use essential oils to create your own natural conditioner without all the parabens, sulfates, synthetic fragrances, and other scary toxins. This recipe is perfect for those seeking a healthy and effective alternative to most commercial conditioners.

10 drops patchouli essential oil
⅓ cup argan oil
Medium mixing bowl
3 vitamin E capsules
⅓ cup non-GMO vegetable glycerin
Spoon
⅓ cup distilled water
8-ounce container with lid

1. Put the patchouli and argan oil in the mixing bowl.
2. Add the vitamin E by gently perforating the capsules with a sharp object and squeezing into the blend.
3. Add the vegetable glycerin and stir thoroughly.
4. Add the distilled water.
5. Transfer to a container with a lid for storage.
6. Shake vigorously before use. Apply a liberal amount to the hair after shampooing and rinse thoroughly.

STORAGE TIP: Store this in a cool, dark place. The expiration on this recipe will depend on the vegetable glycerin and argan oil.

Staying Power Hair Sculpting Wax

Scent: REFRESHING AND HERBACEOUS *Makes:* ABOUT 8 OUNCES
Topical Application: SAFE FOR AGES 10+

Like so many commercial hair products, hair gels and sculpting waxes contain various synthetic ingredients. You can create your own hair sculpting wax at home that controls hair while nourishing it. A heavenly combination of rosemary and peppermint essential oils makes this recipe truly special.

2 tablespoons
   beeswax pellets
Double boiler
Small mixing bowl
10 drops rosemary
   essential oil
8 drops peppermint
   essential oil
2 tablespoons +
   2 teaspoons
   avocado oil
Spoon
2 tablespoons non-GMO
   vegetable glycerin
1 teaspoon
   arrowroot flour
1 small container
   with lid

1. Put the beeswax pellets in a double boiler and heat over medium heat. Remove from heat when melted, about 15 minutes.

2. Transfer the beeswax to the mixing bowl and quickly add the essential oils and avocado oil. Mix well.

3. Place the oil mixture in the freezer for about 20 minutes, or until it has just begun to harden. (It should be more of a solid than a liquid but should still be soft enough to stir in the remaining ingredients without too much trouble.)

4. Remove from the freezer and add the vegetable glycerin. Blend thoroughly.

5. Add the arrowroot flour and mix well. Spoon the mixture into a container with a lid for storage.

6. Apply a pea-size amount to the hair to style. Rub the sculpting wax between your fingers to get out any clumps before applying it to the hair.

Damage Destroyer Detox Mask for Overtreated Hair

Scent: FLORAL *Makes:* 2 TABLESPOONS
Topical Application: SAFE FOR AGES 6+

Many of us treat our hair with not-so-natural ingredients and chemicals when we color it. In addition, many get hair treatments like perms and blowouts that look great but can be bad for our hair in the long run. Hair can also sustain damage from the frequent application of heat from blow-dryers and flat irons. When your hair has had enough, it may exhibit signs of stress such as breakage, brittleness, dryness, and split ends. Reinvigorate your strands with this detox mask for overtreated hair.

½ tablespoon avocado oil

½ tablespoon castor oil

Small mixing bowl

Spoon

8 drops lavender essential oil

1 tablespoon bentonite clay

1. Put the avocado oil and castor oil in the mixing bowl and stir.

2. Add the lavender essential oil and blend thoroughly.

3. Stir in the bentonite clay.

4. Apply the mask to your hair, focusing on damaged areas. Leave the mask on for 20 to 30 minutes before shampooing as usual.

5. Repeat up to twice weekly for best results.

Chapped Lips Rescue

Scent: EARTHY AND FLORAL *Makes:* AROUND 14 TUBES
Topical Application: SAFE FOR AGES 5+

Dry weather can be especially hard on your lips, especially in the winter months. If your lips are frequently chapped, try this soothing and hydrating recipe with frankincense and geranium essential oils.

3 teaspoons beeswax pellets
3 teaspoons shea butter
Double boiler
6 teaspoons avocado oil
6 drops frankincense essential oil
6 drops geranium essential oil
Spoon
14 to 16 empty lip balm tubes or a 2-ounce container with lid

1. Put the beeswax pellets and shea butter in a double boiler and heat over medium heat. Melt until combined, about 15 minutes. Remove from heat.

2. Add the avocado oil and essential oils. Mix well.

3. Pour into the container(s) and allow to set for several hours.

4. Use as needed for the treatment of chapped lips.

STORAGE TIP: Always store salves, balms, and other beeswax-based recipes in a cool place. If they get too warm, they could melt and make a mess.

Winter Lip Protection

Scent: CITRUSY AND FLORAL *Makes:* AROUND 14 TUBES
Topical Application: SAFE FOR AGES 5+

If you are prone to chapped lips, this recipe is great for helping prevent chapping by coating and nourishing the lips. Uplifting lemongrass and lavender combine to soothe and protect lips while creating a wonderful scent.

3 teaspoons
    beeswax pellets

3 teaspoons shea butter

Double boiler

6 teaspoons castor oil

6 drops lemongrass
    essential oil

5 drops lavender
    essential oil

Spoon

14 to 16 empty lip balm
    tubes or a 2-ounce
    container with lid

1. Put the beeswax pellets and shea butter in a double boiler and heat over medium. Melt until combined, about 15 minutes. Remove from heat.

2. Add the castor oil and essential oils. Mix well.

3. Pour into the container(s) and let set for several hours.

4. Use as needed for the prevention and treatment of chapped lips.

SWAP: Frankincense essential oil is a great substitute for either essential oil in this recipe.

Luxurious Lips Sugar Scrub

Scent: EARTHY *Makes:* 1 TABLESPOON
Topical Application: SAFE FOR AGES 10+

Lip scrubs are especially helpful for promoting soft, smooth lips. This recipe contains patchouli essential oil, which is known for its therapeutic effects on the skin. You can look forward to wearing your boldest shade of lipstick after this luxurious lip treatment.

3 drops patchouli essential oil
½ tablespoon jojoba oil
1-ounce container with lid
¾ tablespoon granulated sugar (more or less to achieve desired consistency)

1. Put the patchouli essential oil and jojoba oil into the container.

2. Add granulated sugar until you are happy with the consistency. It needs to be suitable for spreading and massaging into the lips.

3. Apply a pea-size amount to the lips, massaging gently for several minutes. Leave the scrub on the lips an additional 5 minutes for extra nourishing.

4. Rinse off with warm water and follow with Chapped Lips Rescue (page 170) or Winter Lip Protection (page 171).

TIP: You can substitute frankincense, lavender, clary sage, or geranium essential oil for patchouli in this blend.

Calming Chamomile Body Lotion

Scent: LIGHTLY FLORAL AND HERBACEOUS *Makes:* 1 CUP
Topical Application: SAFE FOR AGES 6+

For skin that is often red, dry, and irritated, a lotion recipe containing Roman chamomile essential oil can be a game changer. This oil is soothing to skin and can help reduce redness and irritation. As an added benefit, this lotion is great for soothing the emotions and promoting calm and restfulness.

1 cup unscented
    lotion base
8-ounce container
    with lid
2 to 3 vitamin E
    capsules
20 drops Roman
    chamomile
    essential oil
Spoon

1. Put the lotion in the container and add the vitamin E capsules by gently perforating with a sharp object and squeezing into the lotion.
2. Add the Roman chamomile essential oil. Blend thoroughly.
3. Massage into areas of the skin that need hydration and calming. Use this before bedtime to promote a restful night's sleep.

TIP: Lavender or clary sage essential oil can be substituted for Roman chamomile oil in this blend if needed.

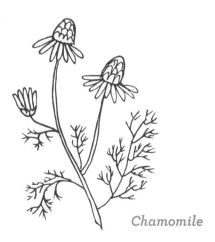

Chamomile

Luscious Lotion Bar

Scent: CITRUSY
Makes: AROUND 10 BARS (AMOUNT VARIES DEPENDING ON MOLD SIZE)
Topical Application: SAFE FOR AGES 6+

This deeply hydrating lotion bar recipe is optimal for dry, cracked skin. A combination of nourishing shea butter and jojoba oil makes this lotion treatment highly beneficial for skin in need of help. Lemongrass essential oil adds a lovely, uplifting aroma.

2 tablespoons beeswax capsules
2 tablespoons shea butter
Double boiler
2 tablespoons jojoba oil
15 drops lemongrass essential oil
Spoon
Ice cube trays or small decorative molds

1. Put the beeswax and shea butter in a double boiler and heat over medium heat. Melt until combined, about 15 minutes. Remove from heat.

2. Add the jojoba oil and lemongrass essential oil. Mix well.

3. Pour the mixture into the molds and allow the bars to cool and harden. Leave the lotion bars in the molds overnight. (The bars will set more quickly if you place the filled molds in the refrigerator.)

4. When the bars have completely hardened, remove them from the molds and store in a cool, dry place.

5. Apply the lotion bars directly to the skin and massage excess oils into the skin as needed.

Makeup Brush Cleaning Treatment

Scent: SPICY AND HERBACEOUS *Makes:* ¾ TO 1 CUP
For Soaking Makeup Brushes to Clean: SAFE FOR AGES 10+

You don't have to waste your money on expensive, chemical-laden solutions to clean your makeup brushes. You can create your own effective makeup brush cleaner at home using essential oils to get the job done right. Clove and thyme essential oils help kill bacteria living on your brushes so you can keep a healthy complexion.

½ teaspoon olive oil

Medium mixing bowl

5 drops thyme
   essential oil

5 drops clove
   essential oil

Spoon

¾ cup distilled water

1 tablespoon unscented
   liquid castile soap

16-ounce glass
   container for
   soaking brushes

1. Put the olive oil in the mixing bowl.

2. Add the essential oils. Mix well.

3. Add the distilled water and castile soap and blend well.

4. Pour the contents of the bowl into a glass container suitable for soaking makeup brushes.

5. Soak your makeup brushes in the cleaning solution for 20 minutes, taking time to swish them around in the solution every few minutes.

6. Thoroughly rinse the brushes with warm water. Allow brushes to dry before using them.

TIP: Make sure the brushes are rinsed thoroughly before using them again. To get any excess oil off the brushes, you can gently rinse them with castile soap before setting them out to dry.

Lay the Base Pre-Makeup Spray

Scent: LIGHTLY FLORAL AND HERBACEOUS *Makes:* 2 OUNCES
Topical Application: SAFE FOR AGES 6+

This makeup primer recipe is perfect for preparing the face before applying makeup. Roman chamomile is excellent for this task, as it can calm the skin and reduce redness. Prepare to look radiant with this pre-makeup base spray.

Small funnel

2-ounce tinted glass spray bottle

1½ ounces warm water

1 teaspoon sea salt (finely granulated)

1 teaspoon aloe vera juice

1 teaspoon sweet almond or grapeseed oil

5 drops Roman chamomile essential oil

1 pipette

1. Place the funnel on the open bottle and pour in the warm water, sea salt, aloe vera juice, and almond or grapeseed oil. Remove the funnel.

2. Add the Roman chamomile essential oil using the pipette.

3. Firmly secure the spray cap on the bottle.

4. Shake vigorously before use.

5. Avoiding your eyes, spritz your face once or twice to prepare your skin for makeup application.

6. Allow your face to dry fully before applying makeup.

STORAGE TIP: Store your pre-makeup priming spray in a cool, dark place. Label the bottle with the expiration date of the first product to expire, which will likely be the aloe vera juice or the carrier oil. To extend the life of this spray, store it in the refrigerator between uses.

Fresh Face Makeup Setting Spray

Scent: FRUITY *Makes:* 2 OUNCES
Topical Application: SAFE FOR AGES 6+

Who needs expensive setting sprays when you can create an effective and skin-soothing spray that promotes healthy skin? Use this all-natural setting spray recipe after makeup application to keep looking your best for hours.

Small funnel

2-ounce tinted glass spray bottle

1½ ounces witch hazel extract

1 teaspoon non-GMO vegetable glycerin

1 teaspoon aloe vera juice

5 drops bergamot essential oil

1 pipette

1. Place the funnel on the bottle and pour in the witch hazel extract, vegetable glycerin, and aloe vera juice. Remove the funnel.

2. Add the bergamot essential oil using the pipette.

3. Firmly place the spray cap on the bottle.

4. Shake vigorously before use.

5. To apply, make sure you have the bottle at least 12 inches away from the face to avoid getting too much liquid in one area, then spritz a fine mist to cover the entire face for best results.

SWAP: Clary sage or lavender essential oil will work well as a substitute for bergamot in this blend.

SAFETY TIP: Bergamot essential oil is phototoxic, so don't apply this spray before sun exposure.

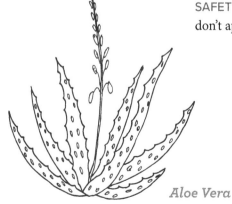

Aloe Vera

Ban the Burn Soothing Aftershave Spray

Scent: WOODY *Makes:* 1 OUNCE
Topical Application: SAFE FOR AGES 6+

Essential oils work to soothe irritated skin, so adding them to an aftershave recipe is highly beneficial. After shaving, skin can become dry or irritated. To combat this, as well as reduce the chances of developing ingrown hairs, you can use this spray to calm and heal the skin.

Small funnel

1-ounce tinted glass spray bottle

1½ ounces witch hazel extract

1 teaspoon aloe vera juice

1 teaspoon grapeseed oil

6 drops frankincense essential oil

1 pipette

1. Place the funnel on the bottle and pour in the witch hazel extract, aloe vera juice, and grapeseed oil.

2. Add the frankincense essential oil using the pipette.

3. Firmly secure the spray cap on the bottle.

4. Shake vigorously before use. Apply promptly to freshly shaved skin.

5. Repeat as often as needed to nourish the skin.

STORAGE TIP: Make sure to label your bottle with the name of the product, as well as the expiration date. This will likely be the expiration date on the bottle of aloe vera juice or grapeseed oil. Store your creation in the refrigerator to extend the shelf life. This also provides a wonderful cooling sensation to irritated skin.

Whipped (Shaving) Cream

Scent: FLORAL *Makes:* 1 CUP
Topical Application: SAFE FOR AGES 10+

Shaving cream can be pricey, and most contain synthetics that can be harmful. Using essential oils and other natural ingredients, you can create an effective shaving cream that soothes the skin—without harsh chemicals.

⅓ melted coconut oil

⅓ cup melted
   shea butter

Medium mixing bowl

¼ cup jojoba oil

10 to 15 drops geranium
   essential oil

Spoon

Electric mixer

8-ounce storage
   container with lid

1. Put the coconut oil and the shea butter in the mixing bowl.

2. Add the jojoba oil.

3. Add the geranium essential oil and mix well.

4. Allow this mixture to cool completely for several hours before proceeding with the next step. (To speed up this process, place the mixture in the refrigerator for about 1 hour.)

5. Once the mixture has hardened, use an electric mixer to whip the contents of the bowl until it reaches a luscious, creamy consistency.

6. Spoon the shaving cream into a container with a lid for storage.

7. Apply a small amount to the desired area before shaving. Massage into the skin and shave as usual.

STORAGE TIP: The first ingredient to expire in this recipe will likely be the coconut oil, but this recipe should have a very stable shelf life and will probably remain good for years (depending on the coconut oil). Store your shaving cream in a cool, dark place between uses.

All Aglow Exfoliating Sugar Scrub

Scent: FRUITY AND HERBACEOUS *Makes:* ½ CUP
Topical Application: SAFE FOR AGES 10+

Sometimes the skin just needs a little exfoliating to look better than ever. One great way to do this is to create your own sugar scrub using essential oils and nourishing carrier oils. This recipe combines soothing Roman chamomile essential oil with beneficial bergamot oil for a unique and therapeutic scrub that promotes glowing skin.

3 tablespoons carrier oil of your choice
Medium mixing bowl
5 drops Roman chamomile essential oil
5 drops bergamot essential oil
½ cup granulated sugar
Spoon
4-ounce container with lid

1. Pour the carrier oil into the mixing bowl.
2. Add the essential oils.
3. Add the sugar and mix well.
4. Spoon the contents into a container with a lid for storage.
5. Apply a small amount to areas of the body in need of hydration and smoothing while showering. Massage into the skin and leave on for up to five minutes before rinsing off.

SWAP: Lavender or frankincense essential oil will also work well as substitutes in this blend.

Calm and Balance Skin Toning Spray

Scent: FLORAL AND HERBACEOUS *Makes:* 1 OUNCE
Topical Application: SAFE FOR AGES 10+

This toning spray recipe can work wonders for skin in need of balance. A combination of Roman chamomile and clary sage essential oils helps calm and soothe skin. This recipe is especially beneficial for those with combination skin. The addition of witch hazel extract and aloe vera juice reduces inflammation and promotes healing.

Small funnel

1-ounce tinted glass spray bottle

1 tablespoon witch hazel extract

1 tablespoon aloe vera juice

6 drops clary sage essential oil

6 drops Roman chamomile essential oil

2 pipettes

1. Place the funnel on the open bottle and pour in the witch hazel extract and aloe vera juice. Remove the funnel.

2. Add the essential oils using the pipettes.

3. Firmly secure the spray cap on the bottle.

4. Shake vigorously before use. Apply an even amount of mist to the face.

5. Repeat up to twice daily to promote healthy skin.

SAFETY TIP: With any blend that is to be used on the face, always exercise caution when spraying or applying to make sure it does not get in the eyes.

Luminous Skin Hydrating Serum

Scent: WOODY AND CITRUSY *Makes:* 1 OUNCE
Topical Application: SAFE FOR AGES 10+

This is the recipe you have been looking for if you want glowing, luminous skin. Essential oils like lemon, patchouli, and geranium work synergistically to promote healthy skin. Skin-nurturing carrier oils make this serum perfect for hydrating and conditioning.

Small funnel

1-ounce tinted glass
dropper bottle

1 tablespoon jojoba oil

1 tablespoon
avocado oil

6 drops lemon
essential oil

5 drops geranium
essential oil

5 drops patchouli
essential oil

3 pipettes

1. Place the funnel on the open bottle and pour in the jojoba oil and avocado oil. Remove the funnel.

2. Add the essential oils using the pipettes.

3. Firmly secure the dropper cap on the bottle. Shake well to blend the oils.

4. At bedtime, apply a small amount to the face, gently massaging into the skin. Avoid contact with the eyes.

5. Repeat nightly for best results.

SWAP: Frankincense essential oil can work in place of patchouli. Additionally, lavender or clary sage essential oil can replace geranium oil.

SAFETY TIP: Lemon essential oil is phototoxic, so don't apply this remedy before sun exposure.

Get the Red Out Calming Spray

Scent: HERBACEOUS AND FLORAL *Makes:* 1 OUNCE
Topical Application: SAFE FOR AGES 6+

Two of the most famous skin-calming essential oils combine in this effective recipe to reduce skin inflammation and redness. Lavender and Roman chamomile are known for their powerful skin-soothing abilities, and witch hazel has also been proven to reduce skin irritation as well. Together, these ingredients promote skin balance and clarity.

Small funnel

1-ounce tinted glass spray bottle

1 ounce witch hazel extract

8 drops lavender essential oil

8 drops Roman chamomile essential oil

2 pipettes

1. Place the funnel on the open bottle and pour in the witch hazel extract. Remove the funnel.

2. Add the essential oils using the pipettes.

3. Firmly secure the spray cap on the bottle.

4. Shake vigorously before use. Apply a thin mist to the face.

5. Repeat up to three times daily as needed to reduce redness and inflammation.

SAFETY TIP: Close your eyes when applying this blend to avoid getting it in your eyes.

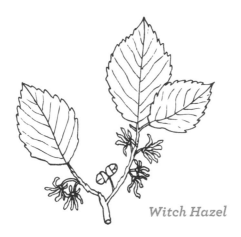

Witch Hazel

Complexion Correction Face Massage Oil

Scent: HERBACEOUS AND FLORAL *Makes:* 1 OUNCE
Topical Application: SAFE FOR AGES 10+

If you are concerned about the look and feel of your skin, this serum might help you achieve a smoother complexion. A supportive combination of geranium and clary sage essential oils can also help promote a more balanced texture.

Small funnel

1-ounce tinted glass dropper bottle

¾ ounce rosehip oil

8 drops clary sage essential oil

8 drops geranium essential oil

2 pipettes

1. Place the funnel on the open bottle and pour in the rosehip oil. Remove the funnel.

2. Add the essential oils using the pipettes.

3. Firmly secure the dropper cap on the bottle and shake well to blend the oils.

4. Apply a small amount of the serum to the face in the morning and evening, making sure to massage into the skin thoroughly.

Healing Oatmeal Mask Treatment

Scent: EARTHY *Makes:* 2 TABLESPOONS
Topical Application: SAFE FOR AGES 8+

If you are experiencing dry skin due to changes in the weather or too much wind or sun exposure, this soothing mask treatment may be just what your skin needs. Oatmeal is known for its ability to soothe skin and reduce irritation. When combined with patchouli essential oil, this remedy can work wonders.

½ **tablespoon castor oil**
6 drops patchouli
   essential oil
Small mixing bowl
1½ **tablespoons**
   oat flour
Spoon
Water (as needed to
   achieve paste-like
   consistency)

1. Put the castor oil and patchouli essential oil in the mixing bowl.

2. Gradually add the oat flour, stirring as you add it.

3. Add water, if needed, to achieve a more paste-like consistency.

4. Apply the contents of the bowl to the face evenly. Leave on for 20 minutes before rinsing off with warm water.

5. For best results, use one of the skin serums in this book after each mask treatment to provide the skin with additional nourishment.

6. Repeat up to three times weekly, as needed.

SWAP: Cedarwood is another effective essential oil that can substitute for patchouli in this remedy.

Time to Detox Mask Treatment

Scent: HERBACEOUS AND FLORAL *Makes:* 2 TABLESPOONS
Topical Application: SAFE FOR AGES 8+

If you feel like your skin needs deep cleaning and detoxifying, this mask treatment is the perfect solution. Bentonite clay can pull out impurities and leave skin healthy and glowing. Lavender essential oil provides hydration and nourishment for skin in need of transformation.

6 drops lavender essential oil
2 tablespoons bentonite clay
Small mixing bowl
Water (as needed to achieve paste-like consistency)
Spoon

1. Put the lavender essential oil and bentonite clay in the mixing bowl.

2. Add the water a small amount at a time, and mix until you achieve a paste-like consistency.

3. Apply the contents of the bowl to the face evenly. Leave on for 20 minutes, then rinse off with warm water.

4. Repeat this treatment up to twice weekly as needed for skin detoxification.

Happy Skin Bath Soak

Scent: FLORAL AND HERBACEOUS *Makes:* 1 CUP
Topical Application via Bath Soak: SAFE FOR AGES 10+

Bath soaks are not only beneficial for our mind and body; they can do wonders for the skin. This bath soak recipe is geared toward promoting smooth, healthy skin. Clary sage essential oil nurtures and calms, while coconut oil helps hydrate. You'll walk out of the bathroom feeling refreshed and lusciously smooth.

2 tablespoons melted coconut oil (or unscented castile soap)
Medium mixing bowl
10 drops clary sage essential oil
Spoon
1 cup Epsom salts

1. Pour the melted coconut oil into the mixing bowl.
2. Add the clary sage essential oil to the coconut oil and blend well.
3. Add Epsom salts and stir, making sure to evenly distribute the oils.
4. Pour the contents of the mixing bowl into a warm bath and let the mixture dissolve.
5. Soak as long as needed; the longer you soak, the better for your skin.
6. Repeat nightly for best results. Follow with a hydrating lotion (page 174).

TIP: Make any bath soak fizz by adding ½ cup baking soda and ¼ cup citric acid to the blend.

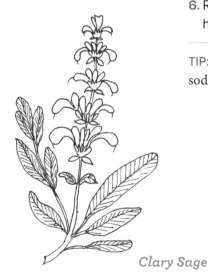

Clary Sage

Family-Friendly Foaming Liquid Soap

Scent: EARTHY AND HERBACEOUS *Makes:* ABOUT 13 OUNCES
Topical Application: SAFE FOR ALL AGES WHEN USED AS DIRECTED

Most antibacterial commercial soaps contain toxic substances that can contribute to the growth of drug-resistant bacteria. In addition, some antibacterial agents used in soaps have been linked to hormone disruption. Ditch the toxic soaps for this effective and long-lasting soap recipe.

Foaming soap
dispenser (reuse a
clean, empty one
if possible)

12 ounces
distilled water

10 drops cedarwood
essential oil

10 drops lavender
essential oil

2 tablespoons
unscented liquid
castile soap

½ teaspoon olive oil

1. Leaving an inch or two of room at the top, fill the soap dispenser with distilled water.

2. Add the essential oils, castile soap, and olive oil.

3. Put the lid on the soap dispenser and shake the bottle gently (not too hard or it'll foam up) to blend the ingredients.

4. Use in the same way that you would use any foaming hand soap. You may need to gently shake the bottle every now and then to ensure the ingredients stay blended.

TIP: To make this soap extra effective, add eight to 10 drops of tea tree essential oil.

Tropical Delight Hydrating Shampoo and Body Wash

Scent: CITRUSY AND MEDICINAL *Makes:* AROUND ½ CUP
Topical Application: SAFE FOR AGES 6+

Essential oils like tea tree and lemongrass combine to create a gently cleansing shampoo and body wash that nourishes hair. The coconut milk is extra hydrating and moisturizing. Replace sulfate- and paraben-filled shampoos with this easy blend.

½ teaspoon grapeseed oil

8-ounce container with lid for storage

10 drops tea tree essential oil

7 drops lemongrass essential oil

¼ cup coconut milk

Spoon

¼ cup unscented liquid castile soap

1. Pour the grapeseed oil into the container.
2. Add the essential oils.
3. Add the coconut milk and stir.
4. Add the castile soap and gently stir to combine all the ingredients.
5. Apply a quarter-size drop to the hair and gently massage, concentrating on the ends. Rinse and follow with a conditioning treatment.

STORAGE TIP: The coconut milk in this recipe will likely expire first, so take note of the expiration date. Keep this in the refrigerator between uses to extend the shelf life.

Stretch Mark Prevention Massage Blend

Scent: FLORAL *Makes:* 1 OUNCE
Topical Application: SAFE FOR AGES 10+

If you're concerned that stretch marks may be making an appearance on your skin, this blend can help prevent them. A skin-nourishing combination of jojoba and geranium essential oils helps condition and prime skin for any changes life may throw at your body.

Small funnel
1-ounce tinted glass
dropper bottle
1 ounce jojoba oil
10 drops geranium
essential oil
1 pipette

1. Place the funnel on the open bottle and pour in the jojoba oil. Remove the funnel.

2. Add the geranium essential oil using the pipette.

3. Firmly secure the dropper cap on the bottle. Shake the bottle gently to blend the oils.

4. Apply one to two dropperfuls to desired areas and massage thoroughly into the skin until all the oil is absorbed.

5. Repeat daily for best results.

Varicose Vein Minimizing Treatment

Scent: FRUITY AND EARTHY *Makes:* 10 MILLILITERS
Topical Application: SAFE FOR AGES 10+

If you are prone to developing varicose veins, this spot treatment can help prevent them from getting worse, as well as reduce the appearance of existing veins. This blend of powerful oils penetrates deep into the skin to target the problem. Remember, bergamot essential oil is phototoxic, so don't apply this treatment before exposure to sunlight.

Small funnel
10-milliliter tinted glass
　roller bottle
9 milliliters (about
　2 teaspoons) jojoba
　or rosehip oil
8 drops frankincense
　essential oil
6 drops geranium
　essential oil
6 drops bergamot
　essential oil
3 pipettes

1. Place the funnel on the open roller bottle and pour in the jojoba or rosehip oil. Remove the funnel.
2. Add the essential oils using the pipettes.
3. Firmly place the roller top and cap back on the bottle. Shake the bottle gently to blend the oils.
4. Apply directly to areas of concern and massage thoroughly to absorb.
5. Repeat twice daily for best results.

TIP: Add two to three drops of cypress essential oil for added healing properties.

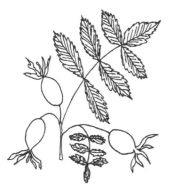

Rose Hip

RESOURCES

Using Essential Oils Safely: www.usingeossafely.com

The NAHA website: www.naha.org

Aromatherapy School and Courses—Aromahead Institute: www.aromahead.com

Robert Tisserand's Website: www.roberttisserand.com

For Aromatherapy Products—Mountain Rose Herbs: www.mountainroseherbs.com/catalog/aromatherapy

All About Plant Therapy: www.planttherapy.com

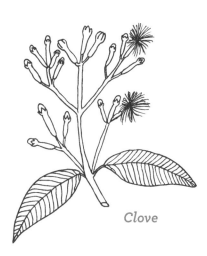

Clove

REFERENCES

Anthony, Amy. "Essential Oil Allies: Patchouli." New York Institute of Aromatic Studies, August 21, 2018. https://aromaticstudies.com/essential-oil-allies-patchouli/.

Anthony, Amy. "Essential Oil Allies: Valerian." New York Institute of Aromatic Studies, October 10, 2018. https://aromaticstudies.com/essential-oil-allies-valerian/.

Becker, Shannon. "Essential Oils to Prevent the Spread of Flu." Tisserand Institute, March 28, 2019. https://tisserandinstitute.org/essential-oils-flu/.

Cai, Shaofang, Jiahao Zhu, Lingling Sun, et al. "Association Between Urinary Triclosan with Bone Mass Density and Osteoporosis in US Adult Women, 2005–2010." *Journal of Clinical Endocrinology & Metabolism* 104, no. 10 (October 2019): 4531–8. https://doi.org/10.1210/jc.2019-00576.

Carey, Daniel, and Patrick McNamara. "The Impact of Triclosan on the Spread of Antibiotic Resistance in the Environment." *Frontiers in Microbiology* 5 (2015): 780. doi: 10.3389/fmicb.2014.00780.

Didymus, John Thomas. "Study: Sniffing Rosemary Improves Memory by 75%." *Digital Journal* (April 9, 2013). http://www.digitaljournal.com/article/347617.

Geethanjali, S. "Efficacy of Clary Sage Oil on Pre-Menstrual Syndrome (PMS): A Controlled Trial." Master's thesis, MGR Medical University (2019). http://repository-tnmgrmu.ac.in/10716/.

Han, Xuesheng, Damian Rodriguez, and Tory L. Parker. "Biological Activities of Frankincense Essential Oil in Human Dermal Fibroblasts." *Biochimie Open* 4 (June 2017): 31–5. doi: 10.1016/j.biopen.2017.01.003.

Jacobson, Lea. "Using Essential Oils Safely During Pregnancy and Breastfeeding." Using Essential Oils Safely. https://www.usingeossafely.com/using-essential-oils-safely-during-pregnancy-breastfeeding/.

Koulivand, Peir Hossein, Maryam Khaleghi Ghadiri, and Ali Gorji. "Lavender and the Nervous System." *Evidence-Based Complementary and Alternative Medicine*, Article ID 681304 (2013). doi: 10.1155/2013/681304.

Moss, Mark, and Lorraine Oliver. "Plasma 1,8-Cineole Correlates with Cognitive Performance Following Exposure to Rosemary Essential Oil Aroma." *Therapeutic Advances in Psychopharmacology* 3, no. 2 (2012): 103–13. https://doi.org/10.1177/2045125312436573.

National Cancer Institute. "Antiperspirants/Deodorants and Breast Cancer." National Institutes of Health. Accessed November 2, 2019. https://www.cancer.gov/about-cancer/causes-prevention/risk/myths/antiperspirants-fact-sheet.

"Parabens." Breast Cancer Prevention Partners (BCPP). Accessed November 2, 2019. https://www.bcpp.org/resource/parabens/.

Sánchez-Vidaña, Dalinda Isabel, Kevin Kai-Ting Po, et al. "Lavender Essential Oil Ameliorates Depression-like Behavior and Increases Neurogenesis and Dendritic Complexity in Rats." *Neuroscience Letters* 701 (May 14, 2019): 180–92. doi: 10.1016/j.neulet.2019.02.042.

Shen, Jiao, Akira Niijima, Mamoru Tanida, et al. "Olfactory Stimulation wwith Scent of Grapefruit Oil Affects Autonomic Nerves, Lipolysis and Appetite in Rats." *Neuroscience Letters* 380, no. 3 (June 2005): 289–94. doi: 10.1016/j.neulet.2005.01.058.

Singh, Ompal, Zakia Khanam, Neelam Misra, and Manoj Kumar Srivastava. "Chamomile (Matricaria Chamomilla L.): An Overview." *Pharmacognosy Reviews* 5, no. 9 (2011): 82–95. doi: 10.4103/0973-7847.79103.

Warren, Ellen. "A Stiff Whiff Can Cut Your Raving Craving," Chicago Tribune, October 19, 2011. https://www.chicagotribune.com/lifestyles/ct-xpm-2011-10-19-sc-health-1019-bit-of-fitness-20111019-story.html.

INDEX

ABOUT THE AUTHOR

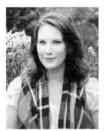

Amber Robinson is a NAHA Level 2 Professional Aromatherapist, as well as an AHG Registered Herbalist. She works with essential oils in an intimate way, teaching the craft of essential oil distillation at her school, The Bitter Herb Academy.

Amber enjoys growing, wildcrafting, and harvesting plants on her farm in the Missouri Ozarks, which she uses to create her own essential oils. She is a wife and mother of two little boys, and loves spending her days teaching them, as well as her students, about essential oils and plant medicine.

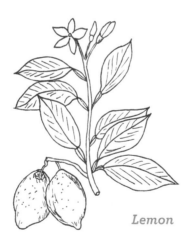

Lemon

CPSIA information can be obtained
at www.ICGtesting.com
Printed in the USA
JSHW011047210420
5206JS00001B/1